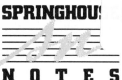

SPRINGHOUSE

NOTES

GERONTOLOGIC NURSING

Mary Ann Christ, RN EdD, GNP

Dr. Christ, a coauthor of this book, is Assistant Dean and Director of the Undergraduate Program of the College of Nursing at the Medical University of South Carolina, Charleston. She earned her BS, MS, and EdD from the University of Rochester, N.Y. Dr. Christ is a member of the South Carolina Nurses' Association and the South Carolina Gerontological Society and serves on the State Board of Nursing's Committee on Revision of the Nurse Practice Act.

Faith J. Hohloch, RN, EdD

Dr. Hohloch, a coauthor of this book, is Professor of Nursing at the Medical University of South Carolina, Charleston. She earned her BSN from Cornell University–New York Hospital School of Nursing; her MA from Teachers College, Columbia University, N.Y.; and her EdD from Indiana University, Bloomington. Dr. Hohloch is a member of the American Nurses' Association, the South Carolina Nurses' Association, the National League for Nursing, the South Carolina League for Nursing, Sigma Theta Tau, and Pi Lambda Theta.

Juanita Tate, RN, PhD

Dr. Tate, the reviewer of this book, is the Division Head of Adult-Gerontological Nursing and an Assistant Professor of Nursing at the University of Colorado Health Sciences Center, Denver. She earned her BS from the University of Missouri at Columbia; her MS from Washington University, St. Louis; and her PhD from the University of Denver. Dr. Tate is a member of the American Gerontological Society, the American Society on Aging, and the American Nurses' Association.

Springhouse Publishing Company
Springhouse, Pennsylvania

STAFF FOR THIS VOLUME

CLINICAL STAFF

Clinical Director
Barbara McVan, RN

Clinical Editors
Lynne Atkinson, RN, BSN, CEN
Joan E. Mason, RN, EdM
Diane Schweisguth, RN, BSN, CCRN, CEN

ADVISORY BOARD

Mildred Wernet Boyd, RN, BSN, MSN
Assistant Professor, Essex Community College,
Baltimore

Dorothy Brooten, PhD, FAAN
Chairperson, Health Care of Women and
Childbearing Section, Director of Graduate Perinatal
Nursing, University of Pennsylvania School of
Nursing, Philadelphia

Lillian S. Brunner, MSN, ScD, LittD, FAAN
Nurse/Author, Brunner Associates, Inc., Berwyn, Pa.

Irma J. D'Antonio, RN, PhD
Professor and Chairperson, Department of Nursing,
Mount St. Mary's College, Los Angeles

Kathleen Dracup, RN, DNSc, FAAN
Associate Professor, School of Nursing, University of
California, Los Angeles, Los Angeles

Cecile A. Lengacher, RN, PhD
Director of the Division of Nursing and Health
Sciences, Manatee Junior College, Bradenton, Fla.

Barbara Tower, RN, MSN, CCRN
Assistant Professor, Essex Community College,
Baltimore

PUBLICATION STAFF

Executive Director, Editorial
Stanley Loeb

Executive Director, Creative Services
Jean Robinson

Design
John Hubbard (art director), Stephanie Peters
(associate art director), Jacalyn Bove Facciolo,
Julie Carleton Barlow, Maria Errico

Editing
Donna L. Hilton (acquisitions), Kathy E. Goldberg,
Patricia McKeown, David Prout

Copy Editing
David Moreau (manager), Edith McMahon
(supervisor), Nick Anastasio, Keith de Pinho, Diane
Labus, Doris Weinstock, Debra Young

Art Production
Robert Perry (manager), Anna Brindisi, Christopher
Buckley, Loretta Caruso, Donald Knauss, Christina
McKinley, Mark Marcin, Robert Wieder

Typography
David Kosten (manager), Diane Paluba (assistant
manager), Joyce Rossi Biletz, Alicia Dempsey,
Brenda Mayer, Nancy Wirs

Manufacturing
Deborah Meiris (manager)

Project Coordination
Aline S. Miller (supervisor), Maureen Carmichael

The clinical procedures described and recommended in this
publication are based on research and consultation with nursing,
medical, and legal authorities. To the best of our knowledge,
these procedures reflect currently accepted practice;
nevertheless, they can't be considered absolute and universal
recommendations. For individual application, all
recommendations must be considered in light of the patient's
clinical condition and, before administration of new or infrequently
used drugs, in light of latest package-insert information. The
authors and the publisher disclaim responsibility for any adverse
effects resulting directly or indirectly from the suggested
procedures, from any undetected errors, or from the reader's
misunderstanding of the text.

Library of Congress Cataloging-in-Publication Data

Christ, Mary Ann
   Gerontologic nursing/Mary Ann Christ, Faith
Hohloch; [reviewed by] Juanita S. Tate.

   p.   cm.—(Springhouse notes)
   Includes bibliographies and index.
   1. Geriatric nursing. I. Title. II. Series.
[DNLM: 1. Geriatric Nursing.   WY 152 T216g]
RC954.T38 1988   610.73'65—dc19 DNLM/
DLC
ISBN 0-87434-116-7

© 1988 by Springhouse Corporation, 1111 Bethlehem Pike,
Springhouse, Pa. 19477. All rights reserved. Reproduction in
whole or part by any means whatsoever without written
permission by the publisher is prohibited by law. Authorization to
photocopy items for internal or personal use, or the internal or
personal use of specific clients, is granted by Springhouse
Corporation for users registered with the Copyright Clearance
Center (CCC) Transactional Reporting Service, provided that the
base fee of $00.00 per copy plus $.75 per page is paid directly to
CCC, 27 Congress St., Salem, MA 01970. For those organizations
that have been granted a photocopy license by CCC, a separate
system of payment has been arranged. The fee code for users of
the Transactional Reporting Service is: 0874341167/88
$00.00 + $.75.

Printed in the United States of America.
SN4-011287

Contents

How to Use Springhouse Notes

Today, more than ever, nursing students face enormous time pressures. Nursing education has become more sophisticated, increasing the difficulties students have with studying efficiently and keeping pace.

The need for a comprehensive, well-designed series of study aids is great, which is why we've produced Springhouse Notes...to meet that need. Springhouse Notes provide essential course material in outline form, enabling the nursing student to study more effectively, improve understanding, achieve higher test scores, and get better grades.

Key features appear throughout each book, making the information more accessible and easier to remember.
- **Learning Objectives.** These objectives precede each section in the book to help the student evaluate knowledge before and after study.
- **Key Points.** Highlighted in color throughout the book, these points provide a way to quickly review critical information. Key points may include:
—a cardinal sign or symptom of a disorder
—the most current or popular theory about a topic
—a distinguishing characteristic of a disorder
—the most important step of a process
—a critical assessment component
—a crucial nursing intervention
—the most widely used or successful therapy or treatment.
- **Points to Remember.** This information, found at the end of each section, summarizes the section in capsule form.
- **Glossary.** Difficult, frequently used, or sometimes misunderstood terms are defined for the student at the end of each section.

Remember: Springhouse Notes are learning tools designed to *help* you. They are not intended for use as a primary information source. They should never substitute for class attendance, text reading, or classroom note taking.

This book, Gerontologic Nursing, uses demographics, theories of aging, and growth and development concepts as a framework for presenting the health problems and special concerns of elderly persons. Such important concerns as legal and ethical issues and income, economics, and health care of older adults are also discussed. American Nurses' Association standards of gerontologic nursing are presented as well as nursing roles and functions. Coverage of health problems uses a nursing process approach; for other topics, nursing implications are listed for all content areas in each section.

Demographics of Older Adults

Learning Objectives

After studying this section, the reader should be able to:

- State what percentage of the U.S. population will be age 65 or older in the year 2030.

- State two factors that explain the large growth of the population age 65 or older.

- State approximately what percentage of the aged population is institutionalized.

- Identify the four most common chronic diseases in older adults.

- Identify the three most common causes of death in older adults.

I. Demographics of Older Adults

A. Population statistics
1. Population of older adults includes those age 65 or older
   a. Young-old: adults in their sixties and seventies
   b. Old-old: adults in their eighties and nineties
2. In 1985, 12% of U.S. population was age 65 or older
   a. Total number of those age 65 or older: 28.5 million
   b. Increase: 2.8 million, or 11%, more than in 1980
3. One in eight Americans is age 65 or older
4. At age 65, women outnumber men by three to two
5. At age 85, women outnumber men by three to one
6. Population of older adults has tripled as a percentage of the total population since 1900 with the greatest increase in 65 to 74 age group
   a. The 65 to 74 age group is eight times larger than it was in 1900
   b. The 75 to 84 age group is 11 times larger than it was in 1900
   c. The 85 or older age group is 22 times larger than it was in 1900
7. Life expectancy for child born in 1982 is 74.7 years
8. In 1987, a man age 65 can expect to live to 78 and a woman to 82
9. In 1985, 2.1 million persons reached age 65, and 1.5 million persons age 65 or older died, yielding a net increase of 560,000 persons
10. Growth of aged population will peak in 2030
    a. Most rapid increase will occur between 2010 and 2030, as baby-boom generation reaches age 65
    b. Growth rate will slow during 1990s because of lower birth rate during Great Depression
    c. In 2000, 13% of U.S. population will be age 65 or older
    d. By 2030, 21.2% of U.S. population will be age 65 or older
    e. By 2030, U.S. population age 65 or older will be two and one-half times what it was in 1980
    f. In 2030, U.S. population age 55 or older will be only age group to experience significant growth.
11. Factors affecting age distribution of population include:
    a. Decreased mortality: premature death from accidents and disease has declined because of improved nutrition, improved sanitation, social improvements, disease prevention, and health promotion/wellness movement
    b. Decreased fertility

B. Cultural statistics, marital status, and geographic distribution of older adults
1. Racial and ethnic composition, according to 1980 census
   a. 89.5% White
   b. 6.6% Black
   c. 2.8% Hispanic

NUMBER OF PERSONS AGE 65+: 1900 to 2030

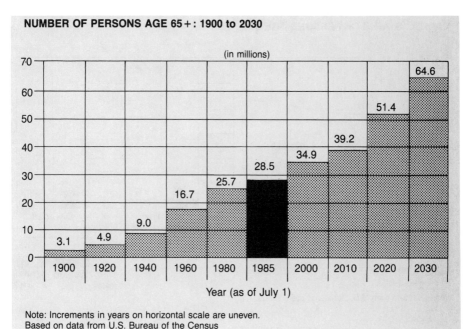

(in millions)

Year (as of July 1)

Note: Increments in years on horizontal scale are uneven.
Based on data from U.S. Bureau of the Census

    d. 0.8% Asian, Pacific Islander, Eskimo, Aleut
    e. 0.3% Native American
  2. Marital status
    a. Men are almost twice as likely to be married as women
    b. 51% of older women are widows; widows outnumber widowers by five
      to one
    c. 4% of older adults have been divorced; number of divorced persons is
      four times higher than it was 20 years ago
  3. Geographic distribution
    a. 45% of population age 65 or older live in seven states: California, New
      York, Florida, Illinois, Ohio, Pennsylvania, and Texas
    b. Persons age 65 or older constitute 13% or more of the total population in
      11 states: Florida, Arkansas, Rhode Island, Iowa, Pennsylvania, South
      Dakota, Missouri, Kansas, Maine, Massachusetts, and Nebraska
    c. Twelve states had more than 10% growth in population of those age 65
      or older between 1980 and 1985: Alaska, Nevada, Hawaii, Arizona,
      Idaho, New Mexico, South Carolina, Utah, Florida, North Carolina,
      Delaware, and Washington
    d. Approximately 71% of persons age 65 or older live in metropolitan areas

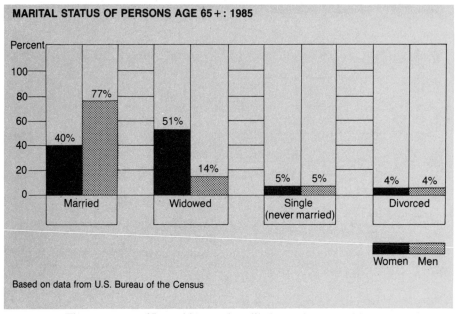

MARITAL STATUS OF PERSONS AGE 65+: 1985

Based on data from U.S. Bureau of the Census

    e. Those persons 65 or older are less likely to change residence than persons in any other age group
      (1) 25% of persons age 65 or older move
      (2) Majority move to another home in same state
      (3) Of those moving to a different state, 42% move to South or West; 25% move to Florida

C. Income and poverty
  1. Median income of persons age 65 or older in 1985 was $10,900 for men, $6,313 for women
  2. In 1985, families headed by a person age 65 or older had median income of $19,162
    a. Whites had median income of $19,815
    b. Blacks had median income of $11,937
    c. 17% (one of six) families had median income less than $10,000
    d. 35% of families had median income of $25,000 or more
  3. In 1985, persons age 65 or older who lived alone had median income of $7,568
    a. 46% had an income of $7,000 or less
    b. 25% had an income of $5,000 or less
    c. 20% had an income of $15,000 or more
    d. Whites had an income of $7,922
    e. Blacks had an income of $5,027
  4. Income stems from various sources
    a. Social Security: 35%
    b. Asset income (income from interest, dividends, rental properties): 26%

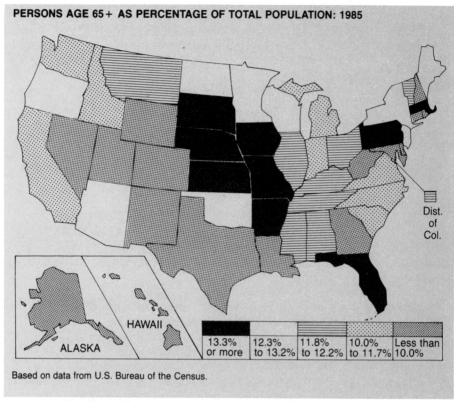

PERSONS AGE 65+ AS PERCENTAGE OF TOTAL POPULATION: 1985

| 13.3% or more | 12.3% to 13.2% | 11.8% to 12.2% | 10.0% to 11.7% | Less than 10.0% |

Based on data from U.S. Bureau of the Census.

    c. Earnings: 23%
    d. Public and private pensions: 14%
    e. Supplemental Security Income, veteran's pension, and other sources: 2%
  5. In 1984, median net worth of older persons' households was $60,300
    a. This exceeds U.S. average of $32,700
    b. 16% had a net worth below $5,000
    c. 7% had a net worth above $250,000
  6. In 1985, 3.5 million people age 65 or older had incomes below poverty level
    a. Poverty rate was 12.6% for people age 65 or older
    b. Poverty rate was 14.1% for people under age 65
    c. 8% of elderly persons were classified as near poor
    d. 21% of elderly persons were classified as poor or near poor
    e. 11% of Whites age 65 or older were classified as poor
    f. 32% of Blacks age 65 or older were classified as poor
    g. 24% of Hispanics age 65 or older were classified as poor
    h. 16% of women age 65 or older were classified as poor compared with 8% of men age 65 or older
    i. Southern states had highest poverty rates

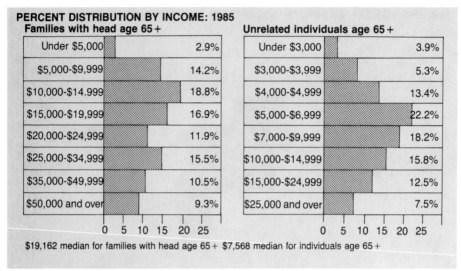

PERCENT DISTRIBUTION BY INCOME: 1985

Families with head age 65 +		Unrelated individuals age 65 +	
Under $5,000	2.9%	Under $3,000	3.9%
$5,000-$9,999	14.2%	$3,000-$3,999	5.3%
$10,000-$14,999	18.8%	$4,000-$4,999	13.4%
$15,000-$19,999	16.9%	$5,000-$6,999	22.2%
$20,000-$24,999	11.9%	$7,000-$9,999	18.2%
$25,000-$34,999	15.5%	$10,000-$14,999	15.8%
$35,000-$49,999	10.5%	$15,000-$24,999	12.5%
$50,000 and over	9.3%	$25,000 and over	7.5%

0 5 10 15 20 25   0 5 10 15 20 25

$19,162 median for families with head age 65 + $7,568 median for individuals age 65 +

D. Chronic health problems
1. Aging and health
   a. Aging is a normal, universal, progressive, irreversible process
   b. Aging progresses at different rates in different individuals
      (1) Factors affecting aging process include genetic background, environment, activity pattern, and nutritional state
      (2) Aging process affects cells, organ systems, and body functions
   c. Young-old population is relatively healthy and active; majority functions independently
   d. Old-old population experiences impact of aging process most directly; chronic health problems increase functional impairment
2. Impact of chronic health problems and functional impairments on older persons
   a. 86% of those living in community go out daily
   b. 88% manage their own care
   c. 79% experience no illness requiring bed rest
   d. 32% of persons age 65 or older assess their health as fair or poor; 8% of persons under age 65 assess their health as fair or poor
      (1) 50% of Blacks age 65 or older assess their health as fair to poor
      (2) 31% of Whites age 65 or older assess their health as fair to poor
      (3) Little difference exists between sexes at any age regarding self-assessment of health status
   e. Most older adults rate their own health as good to excellent compared with others their age
   f. Less than 5% reside in institutions
   g. Four of five have one or more chronic health problems
   h. 86% have multiple chronic conditions

    i. 14% of noninstitutionalized persons age 65 or older have restricted mobility

    j. 12% can't manage self-care independently

    k. Limitation of activities is the major consequence of chronic and acute health problems

        (1) In 1984, older adults averaged 32 restricted days per year

        (2) 15 (42%) of 32 restricted days were spent in bed

    l. Nursing home residents are usually age 85 or older, female, white, and widowed; one in four persons over age 65 will spend some time in a nursing home

3. Chronic conditions affecting health

    a. Chronic illness is major health problem of older adults; most have at least one chronic condition

    b. Physical health problems include arthritis (53%), hypertension (42%), hearing impairment (40%), heart conditions (34%), cataracts (23%), and other vision impairment (14%)

        (1) Women have higher rates of all chronic diseases except hearing disorders

        (2) Poor have highest rate of all chronic diseases listed

    c. Mental health problems include alcoholism, Alzheimer's disease and other dementias, suicide, and depression

    d. The 10 leading causes of death among older adults are:

        (1) Heart disease

        (2) Cancer

        (3) Cerebrovascular disease

        (4) Influenza and pneumonia

        (5) Arteriosclerosis

        (6) Diabetes mellitus

        (7) Accidents

        (8) Bronchitis, emphysema, asthma

        (9) Cirrhosis of the liver

        (10) Nephritis and nephrosis

    e. The 10 leading causes of death in men age 65 or older are:

        (1) Heart disease

        (2) Cancer

        (3) Cerebrovascular disease

        (4) Influenza and pneumonia

        (5) Bronchitis, emphysema, asthma

        (6) Accidents

        (7) Arteriosclerosis

        (8) Diabetes mellitus

        (9) Cirrhosis of the liver

        (10) Suicide

    f. The 10 leading causes of death in women age 65 or older are:

        (1) Heart disease

        (2) Cancer

(3) Cerebrovascular disease
(4) Influenza and pneumonia
(5) Arteriosclerosis
(6) Diabetes mellitus
(7) Accidents
(8) Bronchitis, emphysema, asthma
(9) Cirrhosis of the liver
(10) Nephritis and nephrosis

E. Frail health and old-old age group (adults in their eighties and nineties)
1. Demographics of old-old age group
   a. Fastest growing segment of older population is over age 75
      (1) Less than 14% of noninstitutionalized adults age 65 to 74 need help with daily activities
      (2) 26% of noninstitutionalized adults age 75 to 84 need help with daily activities
      (3) 48% of noninstitutionalized adults age 85 and older need help with with daily activities
      (4) They may be referred to as frail elderly
   b. 40% of nursing home residents are over age 85
   c. Old-old persons in frail health have more and longer hospital stays
   d. They spend more money on health care and drugs
   e. They visit doctor more frequently
   f. Old-old persons in frail health occupy more nursing home beds than hospital beds
2. Characteristics of old-old age group in frail health
   a. Advanced age: 85 or older
   b. Poor mental and physical health
   c. Low income
   d. Predominantly female
   e. Low socioeconomic status
   f. Isolated living conditions
   g. Certain ethnic origins; e.g., Blacks and Hispanics
3. Factors contributing to frail health
   a. Some cannot be changed; e.g., sex, ethnic group, and age
   b. Causes of some factors, such as Alzheimer's disease, remain unknown
   c. Some factors, such as diet and exercise, reflect life-style
4. Impact on health and nursing care of old-old persons in frail health
   a. They are most vulnerable to physical and mental impairment, and experience greatest dependency
   b. They may need basic support for meeting food, clothing, shelter, personal, medical, and financial needs, including
      (1) Physical activities of daily living (ADLs): toileting, feeding, dressing, ambulating, and bathing
      (2) Instrumental activities of daily living: telephoning, shopping, preparing meals, cleaning house, doing laundry, obtaining transportation, taking medication, managing finances

    c. Needs of those persons not institutionalized are met through personal, family, and community resources: day care, neighborhood support groups, nursing centers or clinics, telephone support networks, foster families, alternative residential care

    d. Old-old persons in frail health are usually sicker than those in younger age groups

    e. Nursing role includes:

    (1) Assessing client's functional abilities, assisting client and family to secure needed resources or institutional placement when necessary

    (2) Working with younger adults to change their life-style to promote health and anticipate health consequences of life-style factors in later life

Points to Remember

Aging is a universal, shared experience.

Most older persons are independent, active citizens who can meet their own needs and live satisfying lives.

Chronic illness usually has a major impact in those age 85 or older.

The older population is the most rapidly growing segment of the population.

The health status of an older adult reflects the interaction between the aging process and health problems.

Glossary

Aging—a normal, universal, progressive, irreversible process that occurs with passage of time

Ethnic—concerning groups of people classified according to common traits, such as religion, culture, language, or appearance

Functional ability—ability to perform the physical and instrumental activities of daily living

Instrumental ADLs—instrumental activities of daily living, such as telephoning, shopping

Net worth—assets minus liabilities

Old-old—adults in their eighties and nineties

Physical ADLs—physical activities of daily living, such as toileting, feeding, dressing

Young-old—adults in their sixties and seventies

Theories of Aging

Learning Objectives

After studying this section, the reader should be able to:

- State three characteristics that a theory of aging must include.

- State one difference between genetic and nongenetic biological theories of aging.

- State how memory changes with age.

- Explain the difference between the disengagement theory and the activity theory.

II. Theories of Aging

A. General information
1. No universally accepted definition or theory of aging exists
2. Aging is a normal lifelong process, beginning at conception
   a. Geriatrics: study of the diseases of aging
   b. Gerontology: study of all aspects and problems of aging, including physiologic, pathologic, psychological, economic, and sociologic
3. Theories of aging must include these three characteristics
   a. Description of aging as universal in all species members
   b. Description of aging as progressive over the life span
   c. Description of aging as debilitative, leading to degenerative changes and failure of systems (all systems may not fail simultaneously)
4. All theories and concepts of aging are interrelated
5. Theories may support or refute one another
6. Biological, psychological, and sociologic theories of aging exist
7. Several theorists have described developmental tasks of aging (see "Developmental task theories," page 24)

B. Biological theories
1. Attempt to explain physical aging changes
2. Define biological aging as:
   a. An involuntary process eventually leading, over time, to cumulative change, resulting in changes in cells, tissues, and fluids
   b. Structural alterations resulting from interaction with environment, leading to degenerative changes
3. Include intrinsic and extrinsic biological theories
   a. Intrinsic theory maintains that aging changes arise from internal, predetermined causes
   b. Extrinsic theory maintains that aging results from environmental factors that produce changes in the body
   c. Genetic theories are intrinsic
   d. Nongenetic theories are extrinsic
   e. Physiologic theories are both intrinsic and extrinsic
4. Genetic theories
   a. *Biological clock:* internal, genetic control determines aging process; a set time to live winds down over time
      (1) Rate of aging differs from system to system within organism
      (2) Some individual cells live longer than organism
   b. Characteristic life spans for species
      (1) Maximum life span is specific for each species; e.g., cats, 28 years; dogs, 20 years
      (2) Maximum life span for human beings is 115 years
   c. *Somatic mutation* (failure or error in DNA replication) included in most genetic theories
   d. *Programmed aging theory*: cells divide in vitro about 50 times and no more (Hayflick limit)

5. Nongenetic theories
    a. *Free radical theory*: increase in unstable free radicals from environmental pollutants alters biological system, leading to changes in chromosomes, pigment, and collagen
    b. *Cross-link theory*: collagen molecules and chemicals alter tissue functioning, leading to stiffness and rigidity of tissues
    c. *Immunologic theory*: lymphoid tissue changes lead to imbalance in T cells and subsequent cellular immune function decrease; this results in autoantibody production and immune deficiencies
6. Physiologic theories
    a. *Stress adaptation theory*: accumulated damage results from stress response activation; stressors may be internal and external, may be physical, psychological, social, or environmental
    b. *Wear-and-tear theory*: after repeated injury or use, body structures and functions wear out from stress

C. Psychological theories
1. These theories attempt to explain aging changes in cognitive functions (intelligence, memory, learning, and problem solving)
2. Cognitive function changes include:
    a. Intelligence
        (1) No general decline
        (2) No decrease in crystallized intelligence, slight decrease in fluid intelligence
        (3) Decline in both types in very old age; drop in intelligence about 5 years before death
    b. Memory
        (1) Primary memory (PM) includes information that is held in temporary storage for active processing; limited storage capacity; no age-related change
        (2) Secondary memory (SM) includes information that is in storage and must be retrieved; unlimited, permanent storage; age-related decline and difficulty retrieving information from storage
        (3) Short-term memory includes components of both primary and secondary memory; age-related decline because of difficulty with retrieval from secondary memory
        (4) Long-term, or remote, memory undergoes minimal change
        (5) Major age-related memory change is a decline in the ability to acquire new material and retrieve information from storage
        (6) Age-related decline in secondary memory occurs when task requires organizational and elaborative processes; e.g., list learning, orienting tasks
        (7) Age-related memory decreases can be minimized by using organization and elaboration techniques, repetition and practice, and self-regulation of pace and individual learning methods
        (8) Changes are affected by environment

    c. Learning and problem solving
      (1) Decline in complex problem-solving ability occurs in later life
      (2) Capacity to retain meaningful information does not change with age
      (3) Changes are affected by environment
      (4) Lack of stimulating change in person's life and tendency for older person to learn only useful information affects learning
      (5) Age-related increase in arousal levels before and after learning situations can increase errors

D. Sociologic theories

1. These theories attempt to explain aging changes that affect socialization and life satisfaction
2. No single theoretical framework on social aspects of aging exists
3. Age is not good predictor of social behavior
4. Social psychology assumes:
    a. Stratification by age is necessary for organization of society
    b. Social structures determine an individual's rights and responsibilities
    c. Aging cannot be fully explained using only biological theories
    d. Social expectations occur over course of life; some remain constant, others change
    e. As social expectations change, new ones lead to changes in identity; e.g., retirement, sick role
5. *Social exchange theory*
    a. Social behavior involves doing what is valued and rewarded by society
    b. Aged person has decreased resources and increased dependency, which lead to unequal contribution to society and reduced power and value
    c. With advancing age comes a decrease in number of roles available in society
    d. Roles change with age; person loses worker role with retirement, completes parental role as children mature
    e. New roles may appear in old age: volunteerism, friendships, grandparenting, possible widowhood
    f. Proximity of other people is critical to maintaining social network
    g. Impact of forced change in socialization patterns is not known; e.g., increased or decreased interaction with others, isolation
    h. Friendship with other older adults helps socialize person to age-related norms
      (1) Norms include those of retirement, grandparenthood, widowhood
      (2) Socialization is age-related process
      (3) Few elderly models or mentors exist to serve as examples
    i. Age-related expectations do not remain the same, but change with time and culture
      (1) Each cohort and generation develops specific expectations; e.g., women's roles have changed over time
      (2) Social and historical events; e.g., Great Depression, world wars, affect expectations

    j. For most older persons only a minimal change in physical or psychosocial adaptation occurs after death of spouse

    k. Need for intimacy continues until death

        (1) Some persons transfer needs fulfillment to friends after loss of spouse; women find this easier to do than men

        (2) Men tend to meet need for companionship by remarrying

6. *Disengagement theory*

    a. Elaine Cumming and William Henry proposed this theory in the 1950s

    b. Progressive social disengagement occurs with age

    c. Disengagement is mutual, acceptable to individual and to society

    d. Other theorists suggest that degree of disengagement varies with an individual's personality and life activity pattern and that level of activity (social involvement) is lifelong pattern that remains constant

    e. Studies have shown that changes in health, energy, income, and roles affect disengagement and activity pattern

    f. One study of nursing home residents showed that residents have nothing to do half the time

    g. Disengagement theory reflects observation of some older persons' decreased participation in society; does not hold true for most older adults

    h. Theory does not include social structure variables; e.g., economy, social organizations

    i. Theory does not take into account diversity of outlook and life-style

7. *Activity theory*

    a. Frances Carp and others developed this theory in 1966

    b. Successful aging depends on maintaining high level of activity; involvement in life found to be associated with life satisfaction

    c. Quality and meaningfulness of activity are more important than number of social activities a person participates in

    d. Studies show that when activities in one area decrease, activities in another area increase

    e. Impact of decrease or other change in activities on development of social isolation is not known

    f. Impact of other aging or health changes on activities is not known; e.g., sensory deprivation

    g. Theory does not take into account diversity of outlook and life-style

8. *Continuity theory*

    a. Assumes stability of individual patterns or orientation over time

    b. Recognizes that individual self remains essentially the same despite life changes

    c. Focuses more on personality and individual behavior over time; does not take into account major societal changes that alter individual expectations and behaviors; e.g., changes in women's roles

    d. Assumes maintenance of activity-pattern preference over life

E. Environment and aging
1. This new area of investigation examines the aging person's environmental interactions
2. It focuses on spatial behavior; territoriality and personal space
   a. Territoriality: desire to establish and maintain control over a geographic area; e.g., identify space or place of one's own, assert rights to keep space
   b. Personal space: distance between self and others; smaller with friends, larger with strangers; increases during stress, varies with cultural orientation

F. Aging theories and nursing
1. No one theory explains aging
2. Different theories help direct areas to be assessed
3. Theories suggest in what areas older persons experience changes, how they make major life changes, and how they may experience stress or crisis
4. Theories provide guidelines for assessing a person's adjustment to aging; useful in identifying health promotion needs
5. Theories can provide for consistent nursing approaches
6. Theories can offer rationale for specific interventions

Points to Remember

No universally accepted biological, psychological, or sociologic theory of aging exists.

Various theories are interrelated and can support or refute one another.

Short-term memory decreases with age because older adults have difficulty retrieving information from secondary memory.

Cognitive functions, socialization, life satisfaction, and environmental interaction undergo age-related changes.

Older persons are collectively characterized by diversity, not by similarity.

Glossary

Cohort—a group of persons born in a given year or period who experience the same life events that affect their view of the world

Crystallized intelligence—cognitive processes and abilities developed through context of cultural meaning, primarily education and life experience; uses experience as a problem-solving base

Fluid intelligence—cognitive processes and abilities that relate to neurophysiologic status; creates innovative behavior

Free radical—a molecule with an extra electric charge, having a free electron

Geriatrics—study of the diseases of aging

Gerontology—study of all aspects and problems of aging, including physiologic, pathologic, psychological, economic, and sociologic

Growth and Development

Learning Objectives

After studying this section, the reader should be able to:

- Name five basic human needs that people of all ages share.

- Define ageism.

- State three ways in which retirement affects the developmental task of ego differentiation vs. work-role preoccupation.

- Name four role changes that occur with aging.

- Name one major factor causing loneliness.

III. Growth and Development

A. Basic human needs
1. Basic concepts
   a. Every human being has needs
   b. How needs are met affects growth and development
   c. Changes from aging interact with basic human needs
   d. Abraham Maslow suggests a framework for prioritizing needs
      (1) Physical needs come first, followed by security, love, trust, self-esteem, and self-actualization
      (2) A person has concerns at every level of needs hierarchy
      (3) With age, concerns about ability to meet physical needs increase
   e. Other needs include:
      (1) Identity: having one's own name, family connections, uniqueness in life history, and body image (changes in stature and appearance may affect self-image and identity)
      (2) Rootedness: having a place in time and space
      (3) Relatedness: having someone to relate to, such as a confidant
      (4) Transcendence: no longer being preoccupied with ordinary, mundane matters
      (5) Understanding
      (6) Usefulness: feeling needed and wanted
      (7) Recognition
      (8) Social involvement
2. Factors associated with meeting needs
   a. Degree to which physical and psychological needs meet and interact with other concepts
   b. Such concepts as intimacy/loneliness, power/powerlessness, independence/dependence, confidence/helplessness, acceptance/rejection, control/apathy
3. Possible nursing implications
   a. Acknowledge and address basic human needs of older adult in planning care
   b. Set realistic expectations based on these needs
   c. Educate older adult about body changes and changes in self-image; be supportive
   d. Assess adjustment to aging, including:
      (1) Self-image
      (2) Growth and self-actualization
      (3) Integration of personality
      (4) Autonomy
      (5) Realistic perception of self and world
      (6) Environmental mastery

e. Establish intervention strategies to promote healthy adjustment to aging; the nurse should help:
   (1) Maximize individual's abilities and resources; e.g., encourage older adult to make own decisions, extend social network
   (2) Facilitate adaptation to changing internal needs and external requirements; e.g., assist older adult with life-style adjustments, changes in income
   (3) Maintain or increase older adult's capacity for responding to personal needs and environmental challenges; e.g., help older adult acquire skills to manage chronic disease
   (4) Ensure that nurses become involved in designing programs and developing policies that address major variables affecting successful aging, including poverty, ageism, and social isolation

B. Developmental task theories
  1. Basic concepts
     a. Developmental theorists describe specific life stages and tasks associated with each stage
     b. Developmental tasks are steps to be accomplished in a process that a person experiences as he grows and matures
     c. Developmental theorists describe what they believe is expected at each life stage; thus, many theories exist
     d. Developmental theories may be interrelated and may support or refute one another as well as other aging theories
     e. Age is a major factor in determining life stage
     f. Behavior appropriate at one stage may not be appropriate at another
  2. Erik Erikson
     a. This developmental theorist described developmental stages and specific tasks, based on Freudian theory, that occur throughout life span
     b. Each developmental stage is characterized by specific tasks
     c. Tasks to be met include biological, psychological, and cultural aspects of aging
     d. Task resolution involves:
        (1) Adjusting to old age
        (2) Believing one's life is meaningful and important
        (3) Integrating one's life to prepare for death
        (4) Recognizing that the past cannot be changed
     e. Last task is ego integrity vs. despair (stage VIII)
     f. Successful resolution of stage VIII promotes ego integration; unsuccessful completion results in despair
     g. Successful aging and completion of developmental tasks results in wisdom
  3. Vivian Clayton
     a. This developmental theorist investigated Erikson's concept of integrity and its ego attribute, wisdom

    b. Clayton defined wisdom as the ability to adapt one's perceptions of reality
      (1) New meaning is seen in past experiences
      (2) Old age is a psychosocial crisis that disturbs old ego structures
      (3) Meaning of life is reexamined
4. Robert Peck
    a. This developmental theorist described tasks related to development of integrity
    b. Successful task resolution requires a person to develop ability to reach higher level of awareness, redefine self, and move beyond self-centeredness
    c. Person may be unsuccessful, unable to let go of previous role or to create new meaning
    d. Tasks are as follows:
      (1) Ego differentiation vs. work-role preoccupation
      (2) Body transcendence vs. body preoccupation
      (3) Ego transcendence vs. ego preoccupation
5. Bernice Neugarten
    a. This developmental theorist described increased "interiority" as task of older person
    b. She defined interiority as growing interest in inner development
    c. Inward focus increases; not known if this occurs because of aging or environmental interaction
    d. Inward focus may also result from internal need for self-actualization or because an age-related change in environment (e.g., retirement) causes withdrawal
    e. Neugarten was the first to develop concept of young-old (ages 55 to 74) and old-old (age 75 or older) groups; others have used her concept with different age groupings
    f. She postulated that a continuity of behavioral patterns develop over time and that stability outweighs change
    g. In her theory, aging women move from relatively passive modes to active modes; aging men move from relatively active to passive modes
    h. Her theory refers to social time clock, set of age-related norms for movement through phases of adulthood (e.g., "right" time to retire); believes older person experiences discomfort when engaging in roles or functions at a socially defined inappropriate time; old age has fewer socially defined norms
6. Lawrence Kohlberg
    a. This developmental theorist described six stages of moral development; postulated that crises of adult life are moral dilemmas that result in moral development
    b. Last stage of moral development is defined as universal ethic principle orientation (development of a personal ethical value system)
    c. Morality is defined by and within a person's cultural values
    d. Questions about personal and social value lead person to redefine self

  e. Most moral dilemmas of old age relate to interpersonal concerns
  f. Moral problems of old age involve the following examples:
     (1) Problems with family, such as giving and taking advice, caregiving and living arrangements, and financial resources
     (2) Problems with societal or legal expectations, lawful behaviors
     (3) Problems related to work or retirement
     (4) Problems related to personal freedom
     (5) Problems with friends and neighbors; involvement in others' affairs, involvement in safety or welfare of others, sexual or alcohol-related concerns
7. Robert Havighurst
  a. This developmental theorist described developmental tasks of adulthood that result in satisfactory growth
  b. He defined tasks as "bio-socio-psychological"
  c. He defined successful aging as flexibility of adaptation to new roles within social customs
  d. He identified six tasks of later life
     (1) Adjusting to declining physical strength and health
     (2) Adjusting to retirement and reduced income
     (3) Adjusting to changes in health of one's spouse
     (4) Establishing an explicit affiliation with one's age group
     (5) Adopting and adapting social roles in a flexible way
     (6) Establishing satisfactory physical living arrangements
8. Robert Butler
  a. This developmental theorist proposed that reminiscence and life review are critical to growth of the older person and to development of wisdom and serenity
  b. Life review is an adaptive function of aging and dying
  c. Reflection on regrets or disappointments is catalyst for deeper self-awareness
  d. Butler coined the term *ageism* to describe discrimination against older persons

C. Developmental task accomplishment
1. Basic concepts
  a. Achievement of developmental tasks promotes happiness, successful adjustment
  b. Achievement helps older person view aging as positive or peak experience
  c. Major tasks relate to achieving and maintaining integrity vs. despair, according to Erikson, Peck
     (1) Ego differentiation vs. role preoccupation; establish valued activities and new roles, let go of work role
     (2) Body transcendence vs. body preoccupation; focus on comfort, activities, and enjoyment, not pain and losses

(3) Ego transcendence vs. ego preoccupation; focus on how valuable life has been, legacy rather than death; develop self-transcending philosophy; accept death; teach others about dying

    d. Developmental tasks also relate to social, physical, and psychological losses experienced by older adults, according to Havighurst

        (1) Developmental tasks focus on reorganizing functions and expectations; changing spending patterns to adjust to retirement income; changing functions in marital relationship during retirement; changing living arrangements to address safety, independence, and physical function; adjusting to changes in body function, ability to perform activities

        (2) If individual does not accept and adapt to changing physical abilities and health, maladjustment results

        (3) Developmental tasks stress need to associate with other older people; to change perception of old age; to become politically involved in activities aimed at improving health and social services available to those age 65 or older

        (4) Developmental tasks lead to reappraisal of personal worth in light of loss of work role; finding a source of self-worth beyond work role identity; using leisure time to establish alternative meaningful activities

        (5) Developmental tasks stress need to face reality of death; require active effort to gain closure of life; stress need to ensure welfare of children; involve drive for self-perpetuation and need to leave legacy; lead to period of critical self-assessment, reevaluation of successes and failures of life

        (6) Developmental tasks stress need to maintain self-acceptance, self-esteem, and positive self-concept while adapting to diminished health, social support, and resources

  2. Factors associated with task accomplishment

    a. Successfully coping with multiple losses

    b. Relinquishing power and capacity: "giving up" or "giving in"

    c. Developing compensatory behaviors; adjusting to change; developing new skills, friends, and roles

  3. Possible nursing implications

    a. Incorporate assessment and interventions for developmental tasks into nursing care

    b. Serve as an advocate with families, health professionals, and society to promote aging as positive experience

    c. Recognize and reinforce positive compensatory behaviors

D. Transitions and role change

  1. Basic concepts

    a. Aging associated with many role changes and transitions

        (1) Role losses; e.g., spouse, friend, occupation

        (2) Role adjustment; e.g., retirement, sick role

        (3) New roles; e.g., widow/widowhood, volunteer

        (4) Relocation

  b. Changes in marital roles
   (1) Division of labor changes after retirement
   (2) Social relations change if spouse dies
   (3) Household management changes
   (4) One spouse may become primary caregiver if other becomes ill
   (5) Spouses may need to renegotiate household roles, leisure, and social activities
  c. Retirement: a major role change
   (1) Retirement changes the way a person manages time and daily activities
   (2) Retiree must adapt to nonworker role
   (3) Others must also adjust; e.g., spouse may view retirement as threat to territoriality, authority
   (4) Retirement alters identity, power, status, friendships
   (5) Retiree may need to find new relationships and activities; men usually have more trouble developing new friendships
   (6) Retirement is seen as beginning of old age
   (7) Income, health, and desire to retire affect satisfactory adjustment to retirement
   (8) Those with more income and education seem better prepared
   (9) Some organizations offer preretirement counseling; possible to cut back on work hours gradually to have retirement in stages
   (10) Older adult may adjust better by beginning postretirement activities before stopping work
  d. Other role changes
   (1) Parent-child role: role reversal increases as dependency of parent increases; increased dependency results in loss of power, status, and decision making
   (2) Grandparenting role: by age 70, most people are grandparents; most commonly a supportive, companionship role; more fourth-generation families exist now
   (3) Independent adult role: this is gradually eroded, mostly because of increased dependency, but also from stereotypes about elderly; e.g., health professionals may view elderly persons as unreliable historians and thus discount their self-reports
   (4) Sick role: multiple interactive health problems from chronic disease result in frequent sick role, little power to negotiate care
  e. Relocation: has been associated with possible change in roles, health, income, and type of housing
 2. Factors associated with role adjustments
  a. Age, sex, culture, beliefs, attitudes, income, health, and past experiences all affect adjustment to role change
  b. Change may be a single event but effect is *interactive* with all areas of life

3. Possible nursing implications
   a. Provide guidance for older person regarding attitudes and expectations, identifying new sources of satisfaction and new roles and activities
   b. Support preretirement discussion of role change by retiree and spouse
   c. Encourage preretirement planning and counseling about income, living arrangements, social and leisure activities, and health care
   d. Assist with retirement planning, which is a key health promotion activity because successful adjustment is crucial for healthy aging

E. Attitudes and beliefs
1. Basic concepts
   a. Attitudes are learned through one's culture
   b. American cultural attitudes are diverse
      (1) They value performance, productivity, appearance, self-reliance, independence, and individuality
      (2) They are youth-oriented
      (3) Attitudes develop from Puritan work ethic, which stressed work, productivity, and contribution
      (4) American culture views human beings as mechanistic (Newtonian physics)
      (5) American culture views body and mind as separate entities (Descartes and dualism)
      (6) Use of national resources and policy development is determined by value that society places on group to be affected
      (7) Society devalues elderly persons; sees them as obsolete, expendable; makes older adults feel worthless
   c. Beliefs affect attitudes and feelings
      (1) Beliefs vary with experience, culture, and religious values
      (2) Many persons fear changes associated with aging
   d. Older persons are most stereotyped age group
      (1) Negative stereotyping of older people occurs in literature, in jokes, and on television; perpetuates ageism
      (2) Poor parental relationship or negative childhood experiences may contribute to a negative attitude
   e. Social attitudes are changing
      (1) Currently society is adjusting its attitudes about aging because of increasing numbers of older adults and development of new roles for persons age 65 or older
      (2) Recently more emphasis has been placed on "becoming" and viewing developmental process as unilateral and old age as culmination
      (3) More humanistic approach is emerging; attention is being given to obligations to others and development of self
      (4) Changes in viewpoint have led to recognition of human beings as open, evolving (organismic model)
      (5) More positive attitudes exist in many younger persons, better-educated persons, and those who have had contact with healthy elderly persons

(6) New roles and increasing sense of self-worth are emerging for older adults

2. Factors associated with attitudes and beliefs
   a. Stereotyped attitudes and beliefs result in myths; e.g., "All old people are alike, poor, sick, incapable of change, depressed, will become senile."
   b. Stereotyped attitudes and beliefs can affect health profession
      (1) All aspects of care planning and implementation; e.g., delay in answering call bells
      (2) Choice of career, job selection
      (3) Salaries; e.g., nurses working in nursing homes make less money
      (4) Policy and program development
3. Possible nursing implications
   a. Examine own attitudes about aging
   b. Educate others regarding negative stereotypes and attitudes about aging and their impact on care of elderly persons

F. Religion

1. Basic concepts
   a. Religion may be source of support
   b. Individuals continue pattern they developed in adulthood
   c. Religion can help define self-worth and identity
   d. Cultural emphasis on religion varies; religion is major force in Black culture
   e. Religion gives meaning to life, helps integrate life experiences
   f. Only 3% of those over age 65 have no religious affiliation
   g. Rituals and prayers offer hope
   h. Older adults may seek religious support from church personnel to help deal with emotional problems
   i. Churches provide social activities, crisis help
   j. Church supportive services involve no cost, waiting lines, or records that may create stigma
2. Factors associated with religion
   a. Attendance at religious services may be curtailed by immobility or transportation problems
   b. Strict adherence to religious practice may require special diets for some elderly persons
   c. Some elderly persons may have experienced the death of a loved one that causes them to become disenchanted or more involved with religion
   d. Elderly persons with a limited income may withdraw from religion because they may not have the money they perceive as necessary to contribute
3. Possible nursing implications
   a. Support elderly person's religious beliefs and practices
   b. Find out what person wants; don't assume person desires religious consultation or wants to participate in service; religion may or may not be person's source of support

    c. Remember that spiritual well-being is as important as physical and psychological well-being

G. Losses
1. Basic concepts
    a. Aging is associated with major physical, psychological, and sociologic losses
    b. Elderly persons have reduced ability to adapt to and compensate for stressors
    c. They experience decreased sense of control and increased dependency because of such factors as loss of decision-making role; impact of negative cultural attitudes; crime victimization; mass media portrayal of helpless elderly persons; status and role changes
    d. They may suffer cumulative loss of internal and external resources, relationships, and roles; e.g., possible poverty, poor housing, poor transportation, loss of loved one
    e. Cumulative losses combined with multiple or chronic diseases and limitations increase vulnerability
    f. Cumulative losses may deplete coping resources
    g. All losses are associated with grieving; must complete grieving process for resolution
        (1) Stages of grieving process include shock, denial, anger, guilt, depression, understanding, and acceptance
        (2) Time within stages varies
        (3) Not all individuals go through all stages
        (4) Stages may not proceed sequentially
        (5) Grieving may last 1 to 2 years
        (6) Unresolved grief results in prolonged sadness and depression, which may be translated into physical complaints
        (7) Anticipatory grieving facilitates movement through grieving process; person can begin grieving when confronted with impending loss
    h. Positive aging allows elderly person to overcome losses
    i. Losses and contributing factors of loneliness, depression, and fear of death are interrelated and may exacerbate one another
2. Factors associated with loss
    a. Loneliness
        (1) Multiple losses create deficit in intimacy and interpersonal relationships
        (2) Older adult needs caring, personal contact, confidant-like persons in other age groups
        (3) Loneliness may be associated with complaints of physical symptoms and sleep disturbances and with decreased survival
        (4) Increased risk of loneliness is associated with sensory deprivation
        (5) Older adult needs satisfying relationship with frequent contact to prevent loneliness
        (6) Not all loneliness can be prevented

(7) Death of spouse is major cause of loneliness

(8) Retirement, poor health, and inactivity contribute to loneliness

b. Depression

(1) Frequency and intensity of depression increase with age

(2) Changes in neurotransmitters, multiple losses, and decreased internal and external resources increase chance of depression

(3) Depression may occur in early stages of dementia

(4) Depression is most common psychiatric problem among older adults

(5) Risk factors include recent major loss, feelings of rejection or isolation from family or friends, feelings of hopelessness, absence of identifiable role in life, and loss of sexual partner or sexual function

(6) Depression is most common psychological result of disability

(7) Depression increases suicide risk; suicide rate of elderly men is seven times that of elderly women; person may actively seek death through overt or covert suicide; 25% of all suicides occur in those age 65 or older; white men have greatest risk; risk factors include alcoholism, bereavement (especially first year after a loss), loss of health, living alone, children marrying and moving away; suicide among elderly persons is *rarely* impulsive act; most attempts are not gestures or threats

(8) Depression may be associated with complaints of physical symptoms and sleep disturbances

c. Fear of death

(1) Death is natural outcome of living, cannot be controlled; denial prevents person from valuing life

(2) Preparation for death can be positive experience; major developmental task

(3) Elderly persons think and talk about death; most others avoid topic

(4) Older adults have less fear of death than younger adults

(5) Greatest fears of older adults include dependency, pain, and loss of function and control

(6) Fears associated with death include concerns about afterlife, judgment, and separation from loved ones

(7) United States has a death-denying culture

3. Possible nursing implications

a. Recognize loneliness and intervene to counteract it and increase older person's socialization

(1) Resources include family support, community programs, pet therapy, and crisis intervention

(2) If person lacks support systems, establish network of neighbors, friends, church, and telephone contacts

b. Support older adult in working through grieving process

c. Find out if older person has considered taking his own life and if he has a plan for doing so; keep in mind that person with well-thought-out method (especially lethal method) is at higher risk

d. Refer those with unresolved grief, depression, and thoughts of suicide for counseling

e. Facilitate person's expressions of feelings and loss
f. Support person to mobilize compensatory behaviors, encourage active participation in life
g. Recognize interrelationship of aging changes and loss of resources
h. Suggest substitute for lost companionship; e.g., new social connections, pet
i. Encourage participation in group activities
j. Involve family members in care plans and activities
k. Encourage reminiscence and life review as way to integrate life experiences and resolve losses
   (1) Reminiscence is thinking about and reflecting on past
   (2) Life review is structured reminiscence of life accomplishments using life stages, recognition that one has lived the best way one could
   (3) Process involves action-oriented intervention
   (4) Process involves allowing older person to talk about self
   (5) Nurses can facilitate and enhance process by helping to trigger memories and by listening with empathy
   (6) Older person may need help in summarizing and integrating meaning into life
   (7) Process involves active recall of unresolved conflicts, accomplishments, and failures in life
   (8) Individual or group approach to reminiscence and life review may be used
   (9) Process incorporates traumatic events and normative crises (crises associated with normal life events; e.g., death of sibling)
   (10) Methods include written or taped autobiographies, pilgrimages, reunions, genealogies, scrap books, and albums

Points to Remember

The ability to meet basic human needs independently decreases with age because of multiple losses and changes in internal and external resources.

Healthy aging experiences provide the elderly person with an opportunity to transcend losses.

Negative stereotypes of aging perpetuate ageism.

Depression is the most common psychiatric problem among elderly persons.

Twenty-five percent of all suicides occur among persons age 65 or older.

Glossary

Ageism—attitudinal prejudice against older persons

Death-denying—failure to recognize death as natural part of existence

Ego integrity—acknowledgement or awareness that life has value and purpose

Peak experience—an experience that transcends ordinary limitations and experiences

Physical Aging Changes

Learning Objectives

After studying this section, the reader should be able to:

- Describe how aging changes in the cardiovascular system affect cardiac output, blood pressure, and heart rate.

- Identify aging changes in the gastrointestinal system that affect nutritional status.

- State aging changes that affect renal function.

- Name two anatomic lesions in the brain associated with aging.

- Describe aging changes in vision and hearing.

- State how aging changes in estrogen and insulin production affect the body.

IV. Physical Aging Changes

A. Changes in posture, appearance, and body composition
1. Increase in severity and extent with age
2. Posture
   a. Stooped forward, with flexed knees, hips, and elbows; head tilted back
   b. Causes for postural changes
      (1) Body proportions are altered; shoulder width decreases, length of chest, pelvic, and abdominal areas increase
      (2) Structural change stems from calcium loss in bones and changes in cartilage and muscles
      (3) Trunk shortens because intervertebral distances become narrower and vertebrae become thinner
      (4) Center of gravity changes from hips to upper torso; affects balance
3. Appearance
   a. Loss of skin elasticity, height, subcutaneous fat, and bone mass changes appearance
   b. Result can be overall bony appearance, sunken eyes, prominent forehead, accentuation of elongated ears
4. Body composition
   a. By age 75, body fat increases 16% overall
      (1) Proportion of body fat (adipose tissue) to lean mass increases
      (2) Lean body mass decreases 15% over life span
      (3) Body fat decreases in arms and legs, increases in abdomen and hips
   b. By age 75, body water decreases 8%
      (1) Amount of extracellular water remains the same
      (2) Amount of intracellular water decreases because of cellular mass change
      (3) Total body water decreases because adipose tissue has lower water content
   c. Weight changes reflect changes in body composition
      (1) Gradual weight loss occurs in men after age 55; loss of 20 pounds or more
      (2) Weight increases in women to age 60, then gradually decreases

B. Structural and functional changes in the integumentary system
1. Skin
   a. Slowed cellular turnover from slow cell reproduction in epidermis and dermis
      (1) Cell replacement reduced by 50%
      (2) Healing greatly reduced
      (3) Pigmentation altered; spotty patterns in sun-exposed areas
   b. Decreased blood supply
      (1) Greatest decrease in blood supply to extremities
      (2) Increased vascular fragility; contributes to formation of senile purpura; more common in women

      c. Loss of subcutaneous fat
        (1) Greatest loss in extremities
        (2) Greater loss in men
        (3) Contributing factor in decreased tolerance of cold
      d. Thinning of skin
        (1) Loss of elasticity occurs
        (2) Collagen bundles become larger and stiffer
        (3) Wrinkling and sagging result
        (4) Thin, fragile epidermal layer results
      e. Increased risk of retarded wound healing and formation of decubitus ulcers because of changes listed above
  2. Sweat glands
      a. Size, number, and function of glands decrease
      b. Skin dryness, decreased perspiration, and decreased ability to regulate body temperature result
  3. Hair
      a. Decreased growth
      b. Reduced melanin production: leads to graying; genetic factors determine onset of graying
      c. Altered pattern of growth
        (1) Men experience decrease in scalp hair, no change in beard, growth of hair on ears and eyebrows
        (2) Women experience decrease in axillary and pubic hair after menopause
        (3) Caucasian women experience growth of facial hair
  4. Nails
      a. Decreased growth and strength
      b. More numerous and more prominent longitudinal nail ridges

C. Structural and functional changes in the respiratory system
  1. Chest structures
      a. Increased rigidity of skeletal muscles, connective tissue, and smooth muscle
        (1) Inspiratory and expiratory muscle strength reduced, resulting in restricted ventilation and decreased vital capacity
        (2) Intercostal and scalene accessory muscles and diaphragm used more for expiration
      b. Increased anteroposterior chest diameter
      c. Increased posterior thoracic curve, resulting in kyphosis
      d. Decreased effectiveness of cough mechanism; anatomic chest changes and altered muscle strength do not produce necessary force
      e. Increased rigidity of rib cage
      f. Calcification of costal cartilage
  2. Lungs
      a. Greatest change occurs in persons age 70 or older

    b. 30% decrease in respiratory fluids affects mucous membranes and secretions of respiratory tract; potential for mucus obstruction and infection increases

    c. Decreased diffusion activity results from changes in elastin and collagen components of lung tissue and pulmonary blood vessels

       (1) Decreased tensile strength and flexibility

       (2) Decreased recoil during expiration

       (3) Decreased diffusion from a thickened capillary basement membrane and decreased number of vessels

    d. Increased apical ventilation and decreased basilar ventilation result in poor ventilation of lung bases

    e. 50% decrease in functional capacity from aging changes results in dyspnea with exertion or stress; functional changes do not occur at rest

    f. Inspiratory reserve volume decreases

    g. Expiratory reserve volume increases because air remains in lung bases at end of expiration

    h. Oxyhemoglobin saturation decreases 5%

    i. PaO_2, $PaCO_2$, and blood pH remain unchanged

    j. Total lung capacity and tidal volume remain unchanged

    k. Lungs become rigid

    l. Number and size of alveoli decrease

D. Structural and functional changes in the cardiovascular system

  1. Heart

    a. Cardiac enlargement occurs in some patients; however, this is not a proven aging change

    b. Myocardial hypertrophy occurs

    c. Left ventricle becomes 25% thicker

    d. Elasticity decreases; rigidity increases

    e. Valves thicken and become rigid

    f. Endocardium thickens from fibrosis and sclerosis

    g. Fat infiltration occurs; connective tissue decreases

    h. Lipofuscin (aging pigment) is found in cardiac cells

    i. Heart rate slows with age; resting heart rate remains unchanged

    j. Ability of heart rate to increase with stress decreases

    k. Stroke volume and cardiac output decrease 1% each year from age 19 to 86

    l. Tachycardia is poorly tolerated; heart requires more time to return to normal rate; exercise, emotions, and fever may result in sinus tachycardia that can lead to dysrhythmias or heart failure

    m. Blood flow to all organs decreases; brain and coronary arteries receive larger blood volume than other organs

    n. Coronary artery blood flow decreases 35% between ages 20 and 60

    o. Delay occurs in recovery of myocardial contractility

    p. Increase in myocardial irritability can result in extra systoles

    q. EKG shows increased PR, QRS, and QT intervals; decreased amplitude of QRS complex; leftward shift of QRS axis

2. Blood vessels
   a. Arterial elasticity decreases, resulting in increased peripheral resistance
   b. Calcium deposits in arterial media increase, resulting in fibrosis and sclerosis
   c. Vessel stretch decreases 50% by age 80
   d. Superficial vessels become more prominent
   e. Aorta and carotid artery become tortuous
   f. Capillary basement membrane thickens
   g. Valves in veins become less efficient; varicose veins or stasis ulcers may develop
   h. Veins dilate, stretch, and become tortuous
   i. Systolic blood pressure rises and heart work increases in response to increased peripheral resistance; diastolic blood pressure increases slightly
   j. Altered distribution of blood flow and increased peripheral resistance cause major physiologic changes

E. **Structural and functional changes in the gastrointestinal system**
   1. Teeth
      a. Enamel thins; teeth become brittle
      b. Tooth loss is not a normal aging change
   2. Mouth
      a. Saliva production decreases: results in dry mouth and decreased taste sense
      b. Number of taste buds decreases
      c. Biting force decreases
      d. Gag reflex decreases
   3. Esophagus
      a. Decreased peristaltic activity and relaxation of lower esophageal sphincter results in delayed emptying and increased risk of aspiration
      b. Increased frequency of hiatal hernia may relate to aging changes
   4. Stomach
      a. Fat tissue accumulates and smooth muscle thins, resulting in delayed gastric emptying and difficulty in managing large food quantities
      b. Pepsin and hydrochloric acid secretion decrease; however, this does not result in functional change, except for decreased absorption of calcium and vitamins B_1 and B_2 (amount absorbed is still adequate)
      c. Production of intrinsic factor decreases; however, decrease is not sufficient to cause pernicious anemia
   5. Small intestine: shows no significant functional change, even though absorption of nutrients may decrease
   6. Large intestine
      a. Musculature weakens; peristalsis decreases
      b. Nerve sensation decreases
      c. External sphincter reflex decreases
      d. Age-related changes, diet, and exercise patterns contribute to constipation
      e. Intestinal cell replacement takes twice as long

    f. Diverticulosis of sigmoid colon occurs in one third of persons over age 60

7. Liver
   a. Decrease in size after age 70
   b. Reduction in hepatic enzyme concentration
   c. Decrease in enzyme response to external stimuli
   d. Marked decline in enzymes of hepatic microsomes that participate in oxidation and reduction reactions; affects drug metabolism and detoxification process
   e. Decreased ability to synthesize protein from liver, even though functional capacity of liver remains normal

8. Gall bladder
   a. Emptying becomes more difficult
   b. Amount of bile decreases, becomes thicker
   c. 40% of adults develop gallstones by age 80 (but incidence is not result of aging process)
   d. Amount of cholesterol in bile increases

9. Pancreas
   a. Trypsin, amylase, and lipase volume and concentration decrease, although concentrations remain sufficient to maintain digestive function; decrease may be associated with poor tolerance of high-fat meals and poor absorption of fat-soluble vitamins
   b. Bicarbonate secretion remains unchanged
   c. Insulin release (see "Structural and functional changes in the endocrine system," page 42)

F. Structural and functional changes in the genitourinary system
1. Kidney
   a. Number of nephron units decreases; progressive changes occur in the glomeruli and tubules
   b. Kidney size decreases from reduced renal tissue growth
   c. Extracellular fluid increases and cell mass decreases
   d. Glomerular filtration rate (GFR) decreases
      (1) Decline begins around age 40; by age 90, rate is 50% lower than at age 20
      (2) Decreased renal clearance of drugs results
      (3) 53% drop in renal blood flow from reduced cardiac output results in decreased GFR and decreased renal efficiency; 50% of residual function is sufficient for renal function
   e. Glucose reabsorption from filtrate decreases by 43.5%
   f. By age 70, blood urea nitrogen (BUN) level has increased by 21%
   g. Urine-concentrating ability decreases, especially at night, from changes in tubular function
   h. Creatinine clearance test (a urine and blood test) should be corrected for age; reduced muscle mass causes an elderly person to produce less creatinine; test is best index of renal function in an elderly person

      i. Serum creatinine test (a blood test) does not rise in proportion to decrease in renal function because of decreased muscle mass

      j. BUN level increases up to 30 mg/dl in an elderly person

      k. Sodium-conserving ability decreases

      l. Acid-base disturbances take longer to correct

      m. Chronic diseases of the older adult, such as atherosclerosis, further decrease renal function

  2. Bladder

      a. Capacity decreases by half

         (1) Increased urinary frequency and nocturia occur in both sexes

         (2) Some older adults void every 2 hours during the day and once at night

         (3) They may need to void 30 minutes after going to bed because of increased renal function when in recumbent position

      b. Bladder shape changes from pear-like to funnel-like

      c. Emptying becomes more difficult from weakening of bladder and perineal muscles and change in sensation of voiding urge

         (1) Retention of large volumes of urine results

         (2) Increased frequency or dribbling in men may result from a weakened bladder or enlarged prostate

         (3) Women may experience stress incontinence

  3. Female reproductive organs

      a. Ovaries decrease in size and become fibrotic

      b. Estrogen production decreases at menopause

      c. Breast tissue decreases; size of uterus and cervix decreases; mucus secretion ceases; weakened muscles may lead to uterine prolapse

      d. Vaginal canal narrows and shortens; epithelial lining of vagina atrophies; vaginal secretions become more alkaline; vaginal elasticity decreases

      e. Incidence of atrophic vaginitis increases

      f. Libido remains unchanged

  4. Male reproductive organs

      a. Decreased testosterone production

      b. Decreased testicular size

      c. Decreased sperm count

      d. Decreased viscosity of seminal fluid

      e. Enlarged prostate gland; may atrophy in very old men

      f. Unchanged libido

G. Structural and functional changes in the neurologic system

  1. Brain

      a. 7% decrease in size from atrophy

      b. Atrophy of gyri, dilatation of sulci and ventricles

      c. Decreased cerebral blood flow and oxygen utilization

      d. Neuronal loss

         (1) Neurons do not regenerate; loss is permanent and inevitable

         (2) Cerebral cortex is most affected; experiences a 20% neuron loss

(3) Lipofusion (aging pigment) is found in cytoplasm
(4) Protein synthesis decreases
(5) Ability of hypothalamus to regulate heat production and heat loss decreases
(6) Senile plaques and neurofibrillatory tangles (anatomic lesions associated with aging) develop; plaques and tangles occur in older adults *with* and *without* dementia

2. Peripheral nerves
    a. Decrease in deep tendon reflexes
    b. 15% decrease in peripheral nerve conduction
        (1) Number of dendrites in nerve decreases
        (2) Changes in synapse slow conduction
        (3) Changes lead to slow reaction time
        (4) Lesions form on axons
    c. Changes in baroreceptors
    d. Decline in autonomic and sympathetic nervous system function

3. Neurotransmitters
    a. Increased level of monoamine oxidase and serotonin and decreased levels of norepinephrine; may be associated with depression in elderly person
    b. Decreased dopamine level; decrease greater in the patient with Parkinson's disease

H. Structural and functional changes in the endocrine system

1. Pituitary gland
    a. Vascular network decreases
    b. Connective tissue increases
    c. No change occurs in concentration and secretion of adrenocorticotropic hormone (ACTH), thyroid-stimulating hormone (TSH), growth hormone (GH), and luteinizing hormone (LH)
    d. Follicle-stimulating hormone (FSH) secretion increases in postmenopausal women; remains the same in men

2. Thyroid gland
    a. Structural changes, such as fibrosis and follicular distention, do not result in functional change
    b. No changes in plasma thyroxine (T4) level occur with age
    c. Plasma triiodothyronine (T3) level decreases 25% to 40%
    d. Metabolic rate slows

3. Parathyroid gland
    a. Structural changes occur, but atrophy or degeneration remain minimal
    b. Experts do not know if aging causes decrease in parathyroid hormone (PTH)

4. Pancreas
    a. Insulin release and peripheral sensitivity decrease
    b. Glucose tolerance decreases with age
    c. Experts do not know if aging affects glucagon

5. Adrenal glands
   a. Glucocorticoids
      (1) Secretion rate of cortisol drops 25%
      (2) Urinary excretion rate drops 25%
      (3) Decreases do not have adverse effects
   b. Aldosterone: blood level and urinary excretion decrease 50%
   c. Adrenal androgens: largest component of adrenal steroids; account for two thirds of the 17 ketosteroids excreted; urinary excretion of the 17 ketosteroids decreases by 50%
6. Gonads
   a. Estrogens
      (1) Estrogen production ceases with menopause; atrophy of ovaries, uterus, and vaginal tissue occurs
      (2) Ability to reproduce ceases
   b. Progesterone: production of progesterone by ovaries, testes, and adrenal cortex decreases after reproductive period
   c. Testosterone
      (1) Metabolic clearance rate and production rate decline
      (2) Ovary continues to secrete testosterone after menopause

I. Structural and functional changes in the musculoskeletal system

1. Bone
   a. Bone loss begins around age 40
   b. Diet, hormonal changes, and physical activity affect rate of loss
   c. Reabsorption rate exceeds new bone formation
   d. Trabecular bone loss exceeds cortical bone loss
   e. Bone loss is universal; greater in women (about 25%) than in men (about 12%) (see "Osteoporosis," page 86)
   f. Bone loss predisposes elderly person to fractures
2. Muscles
   a. Muscle cells are lost and not replaced; remaining cells atrophy; total muscle mass decreases
   b. Proportion of muscle weight to body weight decreases
   c. Degree of muscle wasting can be observed on dorsum of hand
   d. Motor unit size decreases; strength declines 10% to 20%
   e. Prolonged conduction time results in slowing of impulses along motor unit
   f. Fatigability increases from changes in enzyme activities
3. Joints
   a. Changes begin between ages 20 and 30; cartilage starts to erode
   b. Synovial membranes become friable; synovial fluid thickens
   c. Intervertebral disks undergo bone loss
      (1) Decreased water content in intervertebral disks contributes to decrease in height
      (2) Degenerative changes cause nucleus pulposus to lose turgor, become friable

(3) Osteophytes form on vertebral column, causing osteoarthritic changes; cervical osteoarthritis develops in 25% of persons over age 50

J. Structural and functional changes in the sensory system
1. Vision
   a. Multiple structural changes result in presbyopia
   b. Lens becomes discolored, opaque, and rigid, resulting in cataract formation
   c. Changes in lens and vitreous humor result in decreased visual acuity
   d. Decrease in depth of anterior chamber and reabsorption of aqueous humor may result in glaucoma
   e. Pupil becomes smaller, reducing amount of light striking the retina
   f. Dark adaptational ability decreases
   g. Arcus senilis appears around the iris
2. Hearing
   a. Multiple structural changes result in presbycusis
   b. High-frequency hearing loss occurs first
   c. Tone discrimination loss also occurs
   d. Presbycusis impairs speech intelligibility (ability to understand another person's speech)
3. Gustation (taste) and olfaction (smell)
   a. Number of taste buds decreases; the remainder atrophy
   b. Sensitivity for all tastes decreases
   c. Experts do not know whether sense of smell also decreases

K. Structural and functional changes in the immune system
1. Thymus
   a. Essential for production of T lymphocytes (T cells)
      (1) T cells control ability to respond to antigen, become sensitized to antigen
      (2) They provide protection against tumor formation and foreign cells
   b. Undergoes involution (progressive degeneration) with age, beginning at puberty
      (1) At age 50, only 5% to 10% of gland mass remains
      (2) By age 60, no thymic hormones are produced
      (3) Response to antigenic stimuli decreases
      (4) Thymus cells become more diversified with age
2. Functional changes
   a. Decrease in natural antibodies
   b. Increase in autoantibodies; results in increased incidence of autoimmune disorders
   c. Decreased antibody response to antigens
   d. Reduced cellular and humoral immunocompetence
   e. Combination of changes reduces person's survival chance

L. Changes in functional reserve

1. Homeostasis requires integration of physiologic, psychological, and social factors to maintain balance; aging changes reduce body's ability to maintain homeostasis
2. As a person ages, adaptive mechanisms may be taxed beyond their ability to respond; deterioration occurs if stress is not reduced and balance restored
3. Physiologic, mental, and behavioral responses to homeostatic stress become more erratic with age and require more effort to restore dynamic homeostasis
4. As a person ages, functional reserves decrease in many systems
5. Stresses within one or more systems deplete person's adaptive capacity
6. Decreased functional reserve and depleted adaptive capacity result in increased vulnerability to additional stressors, including illness, psychological stress, and environmental change

Points to Remember

Aging changes affect all cells, organs, and systems.

Changes within one system may not have major health consequences.

The cumulative impact of aging changes decreases a person's ability to meet functional needs.

Body systems that can meet basic needs may fail to compensate when stressed.

Glossary

Antibody—an immunoglobulin that has the capacity to react with an antigen

Antigen—substance that elicits an immunologic response

Arcus senilis—glossy white line encircling the periphery of the iris, either partially or completely

Creatinine—end product of creatine metabolism; circulates in the blood and is commonly found in muscle; is filtered by the kidney and excreted in urine

Dementia—deterioration of loss of intellectual faculties, reasoning power, and memory

Glomerular filtration rate—the amount of plasma filtrate that passes through the glomerulus of both kidneys each minute

Presbycusis—age-related change in hearing; involves decrease in hearing acuity, auditory threshold, pitch and tone discrimination, and speech intelligibility (ability to understand another person's speech)

Presbyopia—age-related change in vision; involves decreased ability of the eye to accommodate for close work

Pathologic Health Problems

Learning Objectives

After studying this section, the reader should be able to:

- Recognize that signs and symptoms of disorders in elderly persons may vary from those found in younger persons.

- Name the most common eye problem of elderly persons.

- Name the most common cause of respiratory disability in elderly persons.

- Identify nursing interventions that help prevent the formation of decubitus ulcers.

- Identify abnormal laboratory or X-ray findings that occur in common pathologic health problems in elderly persons.

V. Pathologic Health Problems

A. Acute confusional states (delirium)

1. General information
   a. Some references, including Diagnostic and Statistical Manual of Mental Disorders, third edition, revised (DSM-III-R), favor using the term delirium for all confusional states
   b. Acute confusional states may progress from disorientation to delirium
   c. Acute confusional states were previously known as acute or reversible brain syndrome
   d. Acute confusional states may develop over a short period of time (hours to days) or over several months (if caused by a systemic illness or metabolic imbalance); they usually evolve slowly over a period of months
   e. An elderly person's brain is more sensitive than a younger person's to body changes during an illness
   f. Acute confusional states can range from quiet disorientation or inability to fully cooperate with care to agitated states with impaired attention, perception, memory, and thinking as well as hallucinations, illusions, or delusions
   g. Hallucinations, delusions, and illusions should not be used interchangeably
      (1) Hallucinations involve auditory, visual, gustatory, olfactory, or tactile perceptions that occur without external stimuli
      (2) Delusions refer to persistent false beliefs that are firmly held even though they're based on incorrect or illogical inferences
      (3) Illusions denote false or misinterpreted external sensory stimuli that are usually visual or auditory in nature
   h. Possible causes of acute confusional states include:
      (1) Infective; e.g., bronchopneumonia, local skin lesions, diverticular abscess, and bacterial endocarditis
      (2) Neurologic; e.g., drugs with a central neurologic action, cerebral arteriosclerosis, stroke, brain tumor, subdural hematoma, and epilepsy
      (3) Cardiorespiratory; e.g., myocardial infarction, congestive cardiac failure, pulmonary emboli, respiratory failure, and acute hemorrhage
      (4) Endocrine and metabolic; e.g., hypothyroidism, hypoglycemia, hyperglycemia, hyperparathyroidism, and elevated blood urea nitrogen
      (5) Electrolyte imbalance; e.g., dehydration, renal failure, and hypercalcemia
      (6) Nutritional; e.g., cachexia and B_{12} or thiamine deficiency
      (7) Environmental; e.g., decreased sensory input, sensory overload, and sudden isolation
      (8) Miscellaneous; e.g., anesthetic agents, surgical or accidental trauma, tissue anoxia, gangrene, and digitalis toxicity
   i. Acute confusional states increase psychological stress and may lead to further mental deterioration

    j. Elderly patients with dementia are especially vulnerable to developing delirium

    k. Sensory deprivation and an unfamiliar environment contribute to acute confusional states

    l. Decreased sensory stimulation during the night in an unfamiliar environment may cause confusion in an elderly patient with marginal cerebral reserve; this phenomenon, commonly referred to as sundowning, is not an acute confusional state

    m. If acute confusion is not promptly treated, permanent deterioration of cognitive function may result

    n. Acute confusional states have a negative effect on both the patient's health and the nurse's ability to provide care

2. Possible assessment findings

    a. Signs and symptoms may be subtle and vary through the day

    b. The patient may be forgetful or disoriented

    c. Ability to shift focus or sustain attention is impaired

    d. Other signs and symptoms include:

        (1) Memory loss

        (2) Disordered speech

        (3) Misinterpretation of reality

        (4) Hallucinations

        (5) Restlessness

        (6) Disturbance in sleep-wake cycle

        (7) Anxiety

        (8) Delusions of persecution

    e. Tachycardia, sweating, flushed face, dilated pupils, and elevated blood pressure may accompany the acute confusional state of delirium

    f. Acute confusional states usually last less than a week

3. Possible nursing implications

    a. Keep in mind that the nursing goal is to establish a meaningful environment, help maintain body awareness, and help the patient cope with confusion and hallucinations, delusions, and illusions, if they occur

    b. If possible, place the elderly patient in view of a window to help him differentiate between day and night

    c. Keep calendars and clocks where they can be easily seen

    d. Determine what the patient perceives from his vantage point; illusions often result from the patient's limited perspective of an unfamiliar environment

    e. Allow an elderly patient to sit in a chair for short periods during the day, which may improve his perceptions of the environment

    f. Be aware that sudden body changes, such as fever, pain, trauma, or the acute onset of an illness, may produce confusional states

    g. If the patient exhibits agitation or unsafe behavior, address him in a soft, calm voice and ask him what specific help he needs; e.g., "Are you looking for the bathroom?"

h. Implement safety measures to protect the patient from pulling out tubes or falling

i. Help the patient maintain body awareness by allowing him to explore, under careful supervision, and identify foreign objects such as tubes or a colostomy

j. Reinforce the patient's identity by using his life history events to focus on areas of competence and promote a sense of self-worth while minimizing factors contributing to his confusion

k. Help the patient deal with hallucinations, delusions, and illusions by verifying statements and identifying facts; describe reality in a slow and calm manner

l. Identify correctable factors that may precipitate confusion after dark, including:
   (1) Fatigue
   (2) Unmet toileting needs
   (3) Increased noise
   (4) Decreased light
   (5) Sedatives and pain medications
   (6) Fewer staff

4. Evaluation: base on
   a. Successful management of symptoms
   b. Prevention of injury

B. Cardiac dysrhythmias

1. General information
   a. The incidence of cardiac dysrhythmias increases with age
   b. Aging changes in the heart, such as fibrosis, loss of muscle mass, increased collagen, calcification, and occlusion of coronary arteries, contribute to conduction disturbances
   c. Risk factors precipitating cardiac dysrhythmias include:
      (1) Myocardial ischemia
      (2) Hypokalemia
      (3) Systemic infections
      (4) Blood loss
      (5) Digitalis toxicity
   d. Dysrhythmias are more serious in elderly persons because of their lower tolerance of decreased cardiac output, which can result in syncope, falls, transient ischemic attacks, and possibly dementia
   e. Depending on their severity, dysrhythmias may precipitate angina, emboli or thrombi formation, myocardial infarction, cardiovascular insufficiency, or death in elderly patients

2. Possible assessment findings
   a. Symptoms of dysrhythmias result from compromised circulation and oxygen deficit and include:
      (1) Changes in mentation, personality, and behavior

        (2) Decreased blood pressure
        (3) Chest pain
        (4) Dizziness
        (5) Dyspnea
        (6) Tachypnea
        (7) Pale, cool, clammy skin

  b. Dysrhythmias may cause myocardial ischemia with its attendant symptoms, such as dyspnea, fluctuation in blood pressure, and angina

  c. Dysrhythmias may precipitate congestive heart failure in elderly patients; symptoms may include dyspnea, fluid retention, and blood pressure changes

  d. Electrocardiogram will reveal specific dysrhythmias and changes in rhythm

  e. Holter monitoring (tape-recorded electrocardiography) is often used to diagnose paroxysmal dysrhythmias that may be associated with patient symptoms and activities

  f. Pulse may be rapid, slow, or irregular, depending on the type of dysrhythmia

3. Possible nursing implications

  a. Keep in mind that the nursing goal is to assess, prevent, and manage dysrhythmias

  b. Assess for signs of hypoperfusion (changes in mentation, hypotension, and diminished urine output) if the pulse is abnormally rapid, slow, or irregular

  d. Be alert for life-threatening dysrhythmias; frequently assess the patient's level of consciousness, respirations, blood pressure, cardiac rhythm, and pulse; initiate cardiopulmonary resuscitation, if necessary

  e. Removing pressure on the neck or avoiding certain head movements may prevent bradycardia in individuals with a sensitive carotid sinus

  f. Expect to assist with treatment of underlying health problems that precipitate dysrhythmias, such as infection and cardiac or pulmonary disorders

  g. Expect to administer antiarrhythmic drugs depending on the specific dysrhythmia

  h. Expect to eliminate substances that may be responsible for dysrhythmias, such as alcohol, cigarettes, digitalis, and other cardiac medications

  i. Correct electrolyte imbalances, which may precipitate dysrhythmias

  j. Carefully monitor elderly patients receiving digitalis for signs and symptoms of toxicity:
        (1) Anorexia
        (2) Nausea
        (3) Vomiting
        (4) Diarrhea
        (5) Abdominal discomfort
        (6) Headache
        (7) Fatigue

(8) Ventricular ectopic beats or bradycardia (irregular or slow pulse)

(9) Blurred vision

(10) Yellow cast to vision or white halo around light

    k. Teach elderly patients who are taking digitalis the importance of having their serum digitalis level regularly tested

    l. Teach elderly patients the signs of digitalis toxicity

    m. Be aware of drugs that may affect absorption of digitalis

    n. Advise elderly patients taking digitalis to consult their doctor before taking nonprescription drugs

4. Evaluation: base on

    a. Successful management of dysrhythmia through drug therapy and treatment of underlying health problems

    b. Assessment and prevention of complications

C. Cataracts

1. General information

    a. A cataract is the development of opacity in the lens of the eye; usually develops in both eyes

    b. Causes of cataract formation include:

        (1) Normal aging changes

        (2) Traumatic injury to the lens of the eye

        (3) Changes secondary to other eye disorders or such systemic diseases as diabetes, hypoparathyroidism, or atrophic dermatitis

        (4) Drug or chemical toxicity with ergot, dinitrophenol, naphthalene, and phenothiazines or from galactose in patient with galactosemia

        (5) Congenital defects

    c. Although the elderly person most commonly develops cataracts from aging changes, other causes also produce cataracts in the elderly person

    d. Cataracts are one of the most common pathologic problems affecting the aging eye

    e. Cataracts develop at different rates in different persons

    f. Ability to adapt to the gradual vision changes varies among people; factors affecting adaptation include:

        (1) State of remaining senses

        (2) Physical environment

        (3) Life-style

        (4) Individual personality

    g. Cataracts increase the risk of, or potentiate, sensory deprivation in the elderly person

    h. Treatment involves surgical extraction of the cataract (usually done on an outpatient basis) with postoperative correction of residual visual deficits

    i. Surgical procedures include:

        (1) Extracapsular cataract extraction (with possible lens implant)

        (2) Intracapsular cataract extraction (with possible lens implant)

        (3) Phacoemulsification

2. Possible assessment findings
   a. Signs and symptoms vary depending on:
      (1) Location
      (2) Size of cataract and degree of opacity
      (3) Presence of other eye abnormalities
   b. "Second sight," a phenomenon in which vision improves, may occur in the early stages of cataract formation because of swelling of the lens; presbyopic or hyperopic vision may improve, and frequent corrective lens prescription changes may be necessary
   c. Glare is a predominant complaint in the patient with scattered cataracts; patient may habitually wear tinted or dark glasses to shield eyes
   d. Vision may improve in dim light when the pupil is widely dilated in the person with a cataract in the center of the lens
   e. A cataract that develops in the lens periphery may not interfere with vision until it grows over the pupil area
   f. Common complaints include:
      (1) Poor vision
      (2) Eye fatigue
      (3) Headaches
      (4) Increased light sensitivity
      (5) Blurred or multiple vision
      (6) Difficulty coping with sudden darkness, bright lights, and glare
   g. Ophthalmoscopy or slit-lamp examination confirms opacity
3. Possible nursing implications
   a. Keep in mind that the nursing goal is to assist the elderly patient in maximizing vision
   b. Encourage the elderly patient to have regular and frequent visual examinations
   c. Expect to administer mydriatic drops to improve vision temporarily
   d. Teach the patient:
      (1) Proper techniques for administering eye drops
      (2) Importance of not allowing the dropper to touch the cornea
      (3) Importance of keeping eye drops free of contamination
   e. Advise the patient to wear tinted lenses to help cope with glare
   f. Assist the elderly patient in planning environmental changes to reduce glare
   g. Inform the patient who will have cataract surgery about the nature of surgery, temporary restrictions because of surgery, and visual outcome to help the patient plan appropriately
   h. Teach the patient having cataract surgery the following postoperative procedures:
      (1) Protect the eye by wearing an eye shield
      (2) Avoid activities that increase intraocular pressure, which places strain on suture line; e.g., at stool, stooping, and lifting heavy objects
      (3) Avoid rubbing eye and lying on operative side

      i. Assess for signs and symptoms of postoperative complications:
         (1) Iris prolapse (bulging wound, pear-shaped pupil)
         (2) Hyphema (sharp pain in the eye)
         (3) Pupillary block glaucoma (pain, increased intraocular pressure)
      j. Assist the elderly patient who did not have a lens implant with adapting to cataract glasses, if prescribed
   4. Evaluation: base on successful maximizing of vision

D. Cerebrovascular accident (CVA)
   1. General information
      a. CVA, also called stroke, occurs when cerebral circulation is interrupted by an occlusion or hemorrhage involving one or more blood vessels of the brain; CVA causes serious damage or ischemia in brain tissue
      b. The risk of CVA increases with age
      c. Conditions that predispose the elderly person to CVAs include:
         (1) Hypertension
         (2) Atherosclerosis
         (3) Mitral stenosis
         (4) Cardiac disorder
         (5) Glucose tolerance impairments
         (6) Anemia
         (7) High serum triglyceride levels
      d. Major types of CVAs are:
         (1) Thrombotic
         (2) Embolic
         (3) Hemorrhagic
      e. CVAs may be classified according to severity
         (1) *Transient ischemic attack* (TIA): involves loss of neurologic function from ischemia that is abrupt in onset; lasts less than 24 hours without residual signs
         (2) *Reversible ischemic neurologic disability* (RIND): resembles TIA but neurologic deficit lasts longer (up to 2 days) before neurologic signs remit
         (3) *Stroke-in-evolution*: begins as a relatively small neurologic deficit that increases over a period of several hours or days
         (4) *Completed stroke*: produces neurologic deficits that remain stable for a long time and do not completely regress
      f. Clinical features of a CVA vary with the artery affected, the severity of damage, and the extent of collateral circulation
      g. If the CVA occurs in the left hemisphere, it produces symptoms on the right side of the body; if it occurs in the right hemisphere, it produces symptoms on the left side of the body
      h. A CVA that causes cranial nerve damage produces signs of cranial nerve dysfunction on the same side as the CVA
      i. CVA signs and symptoms may be obvious or subtle in the elderly person

j. Recovery from CVA is a three-stage process:
(1) Cerebral edema resolves within 4 weeks
(2) Circulation returns to ischemic areas with some possible neurologic improvement within 12 weeks
(3) Healthy neurons may compensate for lost function, accounting for improvement 6 months after CVA
k. Patient with right-sided hemiplegia may be able to live independently with rehabilitation after CVA
l. Patient with left-sided hemiplegia may not be able to maintain an independent life-style because of spatial and perceptual deficits
2. Possible assessment findings
a. Signs and symptoms vary widely and may be subtle
b. TIA signs and symptoms may include:
(1) Paresis or paralysis of the face or extremities
(2) Aphasia
(3) Vision loss in one eye or hemianopia
(4) Areas of anesthesia
(5) Behavioral or mental changes, including confusion, memory loss
(6) Loss of postural tone
(7) Vertigo
(8) Vomiting
(9) Dysarthria
(10) Perioral numbness
(11) Visual blurring
(12) Diplopia
c. At the onset of a CVA, the patient may become unconscious with stertorous respirations or a Cheyne-Stokes rhythm; pulse rate slows with an elevated blood pressure; if facial paralysis occurs, one cheek inflates rhythmically with respiration; hands and eyes may turn toward injured side of brain; swallowing reflex may be absent; deep reflexes may be absent in paralyzed limbs
d. CVA signs and symptoms may include:
(1) Hemiplegia
(2) Quadriplegia
(3) Hemianopia
(4) Urinary and fecal incontinence
(5) Sensory losses or alterations
(6) Dysphasia
(7) Dysphagia
e. CVA may affect the following seven functions (severity of deficit depends on whether left or right brain hemisphere is involved)
(1) *Language*: with left-sided hemiplegia, language abilities are usually intact; the patient with right-sided hemiplegia may have varying degrees of both receptive and expressive aphasia
(2) *Speech*: dysarthria may be present because of impaired coordination of muscles of speech, usually from nerve damage; the patient with left-

sided hemiplegia may have difficulty speaking clearly; however, he experiences no difficulty in choosing words or understanding speech; the patient with right-sided hemiplegia may have difficulty finding the correct words in addition to having difficulty speaking

(3) *Sensation*: in both right-sided and left-sided hemiplegia, awareness of painful stimuli and temperature may decrease; deep pain sensation usually remains; proprioception may diminish; vision also may be affected; homonymous hemianopia may occur on the same side as the hemiplegia, or the patient may not be able to see out of either eye in the direction of the paralyzed side

(4) *Perception*: the left-sided hemiplegic patient may lack awareness of the left side of body and the environment to the left, with or without visual field deficit; the left-sided hemiplegic patient may ignore stimuli from the left side of body (unilateral neglect); the left-sided hemiplegic patient may have difficulty correctly judging depth and vertical and horizontal orientation in the environment; the right-sided hemiplegic patient usually has normal awareness of body and spatial orientation

(5) *Movement*: paralysis of one side of the body may occur; immediately following a stroke, the affected side may become flaccid or limp; if paralysis does not remit, the affected side gradually becomes spastic or stiff; facial asymmetry may result; if vocalization muscles are involved, unclear speech and dysphasia may result; loss of ability to carry out purposeful, learned motor activity (apraxia) may occur; the patient with left-sided hemiplegia usually develops apraxia on the affected side; the right-sided hemiplegic patient is, in many cases, less apraxic but typically has bilateral apraxia

(6) *Behavioral style*: prestroke personality is an important factor in how the patient reacts to a CVA; usually the patient with left-sided hemiplegia tends to overestimate his abilities and reacts quickly and impulsively, attention span is impaired with poor concentration, concern about disabilities and future develop; the patient with right-sided hemiplegia does not have impaired judgment but, in many cases, underestimates abilities; in both left- and right-sided hemiplegic patients increased emotional lability occurs, characterized by inappropriate laughter or crying

(7) *Memory*: the left-sided hemiplegic patient may have difficulty remembering new information about the environment, such as where the call bell is attached; the patient with right-sided hemiplegia may have difficulty with new language information, such as remembering names

f. The CVA patient goes through the grieving process in coping with loss of function; grieving may be recurrent (note that the patient with left-sided hemiplegia may neglect his left side because of lack of awareness and not necessarily because of denial of his condition)

g. Computed tomography scan indicates evidence of thrombotic, embolic, or hemorrhagic CVA or cerebral edema

    h. Brain scan indicates ischemic areas (may not be positive for up to 2 weeks after CVA)

    i. Other supporting tests include:

      (1) Lumbar puncture: cerebrospinal fluid may be bloody in hemorrhagic strokes

      (2) Ophthalmoscopy: may indicate signs of hypertension and atherosclerotic changes in retinal arteries

      (3) Angiography: may indicate site of occlusion or rupture of blood vessel

      (4) EEG: may help localize the damaged area

3. Possible nursing implications

    a. Keep in mind that the nursing goal is to prevent deterioration of the patient's condition, to maximize functional abilities, and to help the patient accept physical deficits

    b. Remember the following nursing interventions during the acute phase of a CVA:

      (1) Maintain patent airway and oxygenation; keep patient on his side to prevent aspiration, suction as needed; an artificial airway and mechanical ventilation may be necessary

      (2) Monitor vital signs and neurologic status; report any significant changes to the doctor

      (3) Maintain fluid and electrolyte balance; administer I.V. fluids

    c. Check gag reflex before the patient receives food or fluids

    d. Administer stool softeners to prevent straining during bowel movement, which increases cerebral pressure

    e. Provide careful and thorough mouth care

    f. Provide eye care with cotton ball and sterile normal saline solution; instill eye drops, as needed

    g. Determine if patient has language problems, speech problems, or both

    h. Incorporate simple measures into nursing care to promote communication of basic needs, such as using a board printed with simple requests that the patient can point to, if necessary

    i. Prevent or alleviate pain as spasticity increases in the affected side through regular passive range-of-motion exercise, proper positioning, and transfer methods that do not put tension on the paralyzed joints

    j. Closely supervise the left-sided hemiplegic patient for unilateral neglect and for distortions of depth and vertical/horizontal orientation to protect the patient from injury and to assist with activities of daily living; consistently reinforce awareness of left side of body and physical environment

    k. Prevent injury to paralyzed limbs by body positioning and exercises that promote symmetrical posture and movement; consult physical and occupational therapists

    l. Provide eating assistance for dysphagic patient who cannot hold up head; elevate head of bed at least 45 degrees and turn head to unaffected side to facilitate swallowing; semisolids may be swallowed more easily than liquids

      m. Protect the patient with left-sided hemiplegia from injury; caution family and friends that the patient may overestimate abilities

      n. Provide encouragement for the patient with right-sided hemiplegia because he is likely to underestimate abilities

      o. Assess functional ability on an ongoing basis to establish realistic, progressive rehabilitation goals

      p. Support the patient during the grieving process

      q. Provide support and education to people in the patient's support system about the grieving and rehabilitation processes

      r. If speech therapy is indicated, encourage the patient and reinforce therapy

      s. Involve family and friends in the rehabilitation process

  4. Evaluation: base on

      a. Attainment of maximum level of functioning after a CVA through rehabilitation therapy

      b. Successful adaptation to physical deficits while achieving and maintaining maximum life-style independence

E. Chronic obstructive pulmonary disease (COPD)

  1. General information

      a. COPD describes a group of conditions that result in chronic airway obstruction

      b. COPD disorders in the elderly person include chronic bronchitis, chronic emphysema, and asthma, or a combination of these disorders

      c. Most elderly persons with COPD exhibit components of both chronic bronchitis and chronic emphysema

      d. COPD is the major cause of respiratory disability in the elderly person

      e. The elderly person with COPD is vulnerable to bronchopulmonary infections, which, in turn, result in many COPD exacerbations

      f. Peptic ulcers, spontaneous pneumothorax, and pulmonary embolism occur more commonly in the COPD patient than in the general population

      g. Risk factors for COPD include:

        (1) Smoking

        (2) Recurrent or chronic respiratory infections

        (3) Allergies

        (4) Heredity

      h. COPD is a progressive disease; rate of progression varies with individuals

  2. Possible assessment findings

      a. Patient may complain of breathlessness on exertion or shortness of breath or dyspnea at rest, depending on severity of the disorder

      b. Fatigue may result from increased work necessary to breathe

      c. Repeated coughing may occur

      d. Patient may have difficulty sleeping

e. Productive cough may occur intermittently; dyspnea and fatigue upon exertion may worsen insidiously with time
f. Anteroposterior diameter of the chest will increase
g. Breath sounds may be distant because of hyperinflation of the alveoli
h. Wheezing may occur from small airway collapse
i. Typical signs and symptoms include:
   (1) Use of accessory muscles of respiration, especially during expiration
   (2) Prolonged expiration
   (3) Restlessness or twitching
   (4) Hyperemia (engorgement of blood in body part) of hands
   (5) Cyanotic or clubbed fingers
j. Scattered rhonchi may occur with bronchitis because of mucus in the airways
k. Pulmonary function studies show reduction in the ratio of forced expiratory volume at 1 second to forced vital capacity
l. Adaptations to COPD commonly develop slowly and insidiously in the elderly person; e.g., arterial blood gas values may show a low PO_2 and an elevated PCO_2 with a pH near normal from compensatory increases in serum bicarbonate
m. Acutely decreased gas exchange may result in abrupt changes in blood gases or pH and central nervous system depression

3. Possible nursing implications
   a. Keep in mind that the nursing goal is to relieve signs and symptoms, prevent complications, and assist the patient with adjusting to life-style changes
   b. Advise the patient to stop smoking and to avoid other respiratory irritants
   c. Teach patient and family about all aspects of treatment plan; include reasons and instructions for each medication and therapeutic measure to prepare patient to assume responsibility for his own care
   d. Teach spouse or caregiver the signals that indicate onset of an exacerbation, an infection, or respiratory failure; changes in mentation and judgment commonly indicate a worsening of patient's condition, requiring appropriate medical care
   e. Expect to administer bronchodilators, antibiotics, and steroids
   f. Be aware of drug side effects and teach the patient about each medication's side effects
   g. Encourage the elderly patient without heart disease to drink 2 to 3 liters of fluid daily to mobilize secretions; humidifiers, vaporizers, and nebulizers may also be used
   h. Perform postural drainage, chest percussion, and vibration to mobilize secretions and improve alveolar ventilation
   i. Be aware that positions used in maneuvers to drain lung segments can be harmful to the elderly patient
   j. Teach breathing techniques, such as pursed-lip breathing, to control rate, depth, and speed of respiration
   k. Teach patient to cough effectively

l. Expect to administer oxygen

m. Teach patient and family the purpose of oxygen therapy, how to use and clean equipment, and signs and symptoms of carbon dioxide narcosis, if oxygen therapy is continued at home

n. Encourage development of an exercise program; usually discussed with doctor; must be carefully planned, graded, and closely supervised

o. Assist the patient in planning and managing life-style changes as COPD progresses

p. Encourage the patient to verbalize feelings and to work through the grieving process while adapting to chronic illness

q. Support and assist patient and family to accept altered life-style

4. Evaluation: base on adaptation to illness and life-style changes as disease progresses

F. Congestive heart failure (CHF)

1. General information

a. CHF is a syndrome in which the heart fails to pump effectively, resulting in circulatory and/or pulmonary congestion; pump failure in the right ventricle is right-sided heart failure; pump failure in the left ventricle is left-sided heart failure

b. Chronic CHF may have an insidious onset because of the development of compensatory mechanisms that attempt to maintain adequate cardiac output and perfusion

c. CHF incidence and prevalence increase with age

d. The elderly patient with CHF usually has at least one other cardiac disease and other noncardiac health problems

e. Common cardiac diseases associated with CHF in the elderly patient are:

(1) Coronary artery disease

(2) Myocardial infarction

(3) Hypertension associated with cardiac hypertrophy and heart wall stiffness

f. Disorders that increase the risk of CHF development include:

(1) Chronic obstructive pulmonary disease

(2) Pulmonary emboli

(3) Renal disease

(4) Liver disease

(5) Hyperthyroidism

(6) Anemia

g. Risk factors for CHF development include:

(1) Obesity

(2) Malnutrition

(3) High-sodium diet

h. Drugs affecting cardiac pumping ability and those causing sodium and water retention can precipitate CHF in the elderly patient

i. Emotional stress and excessive or insufficient physical activity are associated with CHF in the elderly patient

j. In many cases, the elderly patient with CHF can manage the condition at home with medications, special diet, and modification of exercise and activities of daily living

k. When treating CHF in elderly patients, special considerations include their smaller cardiac reserve and increased risk of such disorders as thrombophlebitis, pulmonary embolism, decubitus ulcers, and pneumonia associated with immobility

2. Possible assessment findings

a. Other disease processes may obscure classic signs and symptoms of CHF in the elderly patient

b. Signs and symptoms associated with left-sided heart failure include:
(1) Breathlessness
(2) Dyspnea on exertion or at rest
(3) Productive cough
(4) Pulmonary congestion
(5) Wheezing
(6) Nocturia
(7) Crackles at bases of lungs that do not clear with coughing

c. Signs and symptoms associated with right-sided heart failure include:
(1) Edema of the lower extremities
(2) Engorgement of neck veins
(3) Hepatic enlargement and tenderness
(4) Abdominal distention
(5) Anorexia
(6) Nausea
(7) Vomiting
(8) Ascites
(9) Renal insufficiency or oliguria

d. The elderly patient may exhibit signs and symptoms of both left- and right-sided heart failure

e. Chest pain or tightness may accompany CHF in the elderly patient

f. Diagnostic tests include a chest X-ray taken after full inspiration to detect changes in pulmonary vessels and cardiac dilation; laboratory tests attempt to identify precipitating causes of heart failure

3. Possible nursing implications

a. Keep in mind that the nursing goal is to decrease cardiac workload, increase cardiac output, and reduce vascular congestion

b. Monitor for signs and symptoms of progressive CHF, such as increased dyspnea, coughing, or edema

c. Remember that chair rest is preferable to bed rest, if tolerated by the patient

d. Observe the patient doing simple activities, such as repositioning in bed, eating, washing, and talking, to evaluate level of activity tolerance

e. Teach the patient to avoid Valsalva's maneuver when turning

f. Assist the patient with applying antiembolic elastic stockings to prevent deep vein thrombosis and emboli

    g. Assist the patient in planning daily activities that incorporate rest periods

    h. Monitor emotional responses to care plan

    i. Assist the patient in modifying diet to meet sodium restriction

    j. Confirm that the patient understands and follows the sodium-restricted diet

    k. Provide emotional support through reassurance and education

    l. Counsel family members and significant others about the need for emotional support and the need to avoid emotionally stressful interactions

    m. Expect to administer diuretics

    n. Monitor for signs and symptoms of hypokalemia or dehydration, such as weakness, dizziness, and confusion, which are side effects of diuretics

    o. Weigh the patient daily at the same time and in the same clothing to monitor diuresis and degree of edema accurately

    p. Expect to administer cardiac glycosides, such as digitoxin or digoxin

    q. Assess for signs and symptoms of digitalis toxicity, such as anorexia, nausea, vomiting, headache, premature ventricular contractions, bradycardia; be especially alert if the patient is taking a diuretic and digitalis

    r. Educate the patient about medication regimen and the importance of continuing regularly scheduled laboratory tests (serum digitalis levels, serum electrolyte levels, and blood urea nitrogen levels)

    s. Advise the patient and family to see the doctor if they notice signs or symptoms of CHF exacerbation, including:

        (1) Shortness of breath

        (2) Coughing

        (3) Edema of feet, legs, and ankles

        (4) Weight gain

    t. Expect to administer oxygen therapy

    u. If oxygen therapy is continued at home, teach the patient and family the purpose of oxygen therapy and how to use and clean equipment

  4. Evaluation: base on

    a. Management of symptoms and decreased incidence of CHF exacerbation

    b. Successful adaptation to life-style changes related to diet, medication, and activity level

G. Decubitus ulcer

  1. General information

    a. Decubitus ulcers (pressure sores) develop from obstruction of capillary flow that leads to acute tissue ischemia, tissue necrosis, and subsequent ulceration

    b. Unrelieved pressure, immobility, and shear forces (friction) contribute to the development of decubitus ulcers

    c. Factors that place the elderly patient at risk for developing decubitus ulcers include:

        (1) Immobility

        (2) Impaired sensitivity to pain

       (3) Paralysis
       (4) Malnutrition
       (5) Impaired circulation
       (6) Incontinence
       (7) Obesity
       (8) Edema
       (9) Anemia
      (10) Confusion
      (11) Warm, moist skin areas

  d. Immobility is the biggest single risk factor for development of decubitus ulcers

  e. Common sites for development of decubitus ulcers include:
     (1) Heel
     (2) Greater trochanter
     (3) Sacrum
     (4) Elbow
     (5) Scapular spine
     (6) Dorsal spine in thin kyphotic individuals

  f. Slow healing because of circulatory inadequacy and the potential for infection make decubitus ulcers a serious problem for the elderly patient

  g. Nursing intervention at any stage of decubitus ulcer development will prevent further ulcer progression

  h. Enzyme products are used in many cases to debride ulcers with large amounts of necrotic tissue and eschar

  i. Antibiotic products can decrease the number of bacteria or fungi in the decubitus ulcer

2. Possible assessment findings

  a. Decubitus ulcer formation can be classified into 4 stages
     (1) Stage 1: skin appears shiny with erythema over the compressed area
     (2) Stage 2: small blisters or erosions develop
     (3) Stage 3: skin is broken, creating a deep pressure sore and tissue involvement
     (4) Stage 4: deep pressure sore with tissue, bone, and muscle involvement

  b. The presence of bacteria in the affected area causes inflammation and further necrosis

  c. Black eschar may be present

  d. Foul-smelling, purulent discharge may be present in advanced stages of ulcer development

  e. Culture and sensitivity test of exudate will identify organisms present and determine appropriate antibiotics

3. Possible nursing implications

  a. Keep in mind that the nursing goal is to assist with measures to heal the decubitus ulcer, limit its effects, and prevent recurrence

  b. Identify the high-risk patient and initiate vigorous measures to prevent decubitus ulcer formation

    c. Reposition the immobilized patient at least every 2 hours, depending on the patient's condition

    d. Use alternating air mattresses and padding to alleviate pressure

    e. Keep bed clean, dry, and free of wrinkles to help prevent ulcer formation

    f. Provide meticulous skin care, especially to the incontinent patient; moist skin and feces predispose area to tissue breakdown and infection

    g. Massage back and all bony prominences (coccyx, hips, elbows, heels, shoulder blades, knees, and ankles) several times a day, especially when repositioning

    h. Promote healing of decubitus ulcers; interventions include:
        (1) Providing good nutrition
        (2) Relieving pressure
        (3) Promoting good circulation
        (4) Providing meticulous skin care
        (5) Positioning properly

    i. Keep in mind that many intervention techniques are used to treat a decubitus ulcer, including:
        (1) Heat lamp
        (2) Chemical debridement agents
        (3) Wet-to-dry dressings
        (4) Irrigations and soaks with various agents

    j. Assist patient with whirlpool treatments to promote circulation

    k. Encourage adequate food and fluid intake to promote optimum healing

  4. Evaluation: base on

    a. Successful management and healing of ulcer

    b. Prevention of further ulcer development

H. Dementia

  1. General information

    a. Dementia involves a permanent, progressive deterioration of mental function characterized by confusion, impaired judgment, forgetfulness, and personality changes

    b. The two most common types of dementia are multi-infarct dementia and Alzheimer's disease

    c. Multi-infarct dementia
        (1) This condition results from repeated strokes that cause complete deterioration of cerebral tissue within a circumscribed area
        (2) Its onset may be gradual or sudden
        (3) Its course is marked by a cyclical worsening and lessening of signs and symptoms
        (4) The early phase of multi-infarct dementia shows a gradual progression of impaired intellectual functioning and partial memory lapses; symptoms include dizziness, headaches, decreased physical and mental vigor, and vague physical complaints
        (5) Delirium may result from insufficient cerebral circulation in multi-infarct dementia

d. Alzheimer's disease

(1) This disease is characterized by brain atrophy and the presence of neurofibrillary tangles, granulovascular changes, neuritic (senile) plaques, and reduced cholinergic enervation

(2) Symptoms appear gradually, beginning with impaired memory and progressing to language and motor difficulties

(3) The cause of Alzheimer's disease is unknown

(4) The first stage lasts from 2 to 4 years and is marked by spatial and time disorientation, inappropriate affect, decreased concentration, transient paranoia, careless dressing or grooming, impaired judgment, forgetfulness, perceptual disturbances, and memory loss

(5) The second stage, lasting up to 7 years, is marked by more profound changes and loss of independence; symptoms include the inability to recognize familiar persons or to interpret the environment, poor comprehension, nocturnal restlessness, apraxia, ravenous appetite but no weight gain, complete disorientation, wandering, asterognosia, hoarding, inability to read or write, communication difficulties, hypertonia, and both short- and long-term memory loss

(6) The last stage occurs during the final year and is marked by a blank facial expression, paraphasia, irritability, hyperorality, seizures, inability to recognize family members, loss of appetite, emaciation, and total dependence

(7) Estimates on the illness's duration vary in the literature from 5 to 14 years before death occurs

(8) Factors that frequently contribute to the Alzheimer's patient's death include pneumonia or other infections, malnutrition, and dehydration

(9) Postmortem brain biopsy is currently the only definitive test for Alzheimer's disease; otherwise, a provisional diagnosis is given after excluding other causes of dementia

2. Possible assessment findings

a. Patients with dementia may deny memory loss or make vague complaints of fatigue, dizziness, or occasional headaches

b. The patient may appear in good health except for memory and behavioral changes

c. The patient may appear fearful and suspicious, clinging to significant others or claiming that misplaced items are stolen

d. Signs and symptoms related to multi-infarct dementia vary with the brain area affected

e. Symptoms may vary and progress at different rates

f. Laboratory tests, such as complete blood count, VDRL test, electrolyte levels, and thyroid studies, are ordered to rule out treatable causes of dementia

g. A thorough drug history rules out drug-induced dementia

h. A mental status examination is performed to differentiate dementia from depression

    i. A thorough physical, neurologic, and psychiatric examination rules out other disorders that may cause similar signs and symptoms

    j. Computed tomography may show evidence of stroke, multi-infarct dementia, tumors, changes in the flow of cerebrospinal fluid, hematomas, and cerebral atrophy

    k. Positron emission tomography, which measures metabolic activity of the cerebral cortex, can be used to differentiate other dementias from Alzheimer's disease

3. Possible nursing implications

    a. Keep in mind that the nursing goal is to help the patient maintain optimum health, to protect him from injury, and to provide physical and intellectual stimulation

    b. Assist the patient with memory deficits by incorporating reality orientation as an ongoing process during all nursing interventions

    c. Reassure the patient who overreacts to unfamiliar situations by speaking calmly and slowly and by reducing environmental distractions

    d. Offer support and recognize the patient's feelings as he tries to cope with the loss of personal finances and independence, employment difficulties, and inability to drive a car or perform simple daily activities

    e. Offer support to family members and caregivers by explaining the progression of the disease, educating them about how to alleviate symptoms, and recommending community resources and support groups

    f. Assist the family and caregivers in managing such problems as wandering, eating, toileting, and inappropriate behavior

    g. Protect the patient from injury by teaching his caregiver to identify and correct potential safety hazards

4. Evaluation: base on

    a. Management of the patient's behavioral and personality changes

    b. Educating the patient, family members, and caregivers about coping strategies and community resources

I. Diabetes mellitus

1. General information

    a. Diabetes mellitus is a chronic disease of insulin deficiency or resistance (resistance renders insulin ineffective)

    b. Diabetes mellitus is characterized by hyperglycemia, insulin deficiency or resistance, and premature degenerative changes in the nervous and circulatory system

    c. Two types of diabetes occur

      (1) Insulin-dependent diabetes mellitus (IDDM), Type I: usually occurs before age 25 but can develop in the elderly person; little or no insulin production

      (2) Non-insulin-dependent diabetes mellitus (NIDDM), Type II: usually develops after age 40 and is commonly seen in the elderly person; insulin is produced but may be insufficient or ineffective in preventing hyperglycemia

    d. Glucose intolerance (impaired ability to metabolize glucose) in the elderly person may occur from age-related changes in insulin levels and insulin release, decreased peripheral effectiveness of insulin, or a combination of these factors

    e. Acute illness increases insulin demand

    f. Decreased exercise levels in the elderly person may result in decreased glucose tolerance

    g. Medications commonly taken by the elderly person, such as thiazide diuretics, furosemide, ethacrynic acid, nicotinic acid, estrogen, cortisone, and levodopa, may contribute to poor glucose tolerance

    h. Atherosclerotic cardiovascular disease may develop prematurely in the diabetic patient

    i. Risk factors for diabetes mellitus include:
       (1) Heredity
       (2) Obesity
       (3) Prolonged elevation of stress hormone levels (cortisol, epinephrine, glucagon, and growth hormone) from physiologic or emotional stress

    j. The newly diagnosed elderly diabetic patient is commonly managed by a low-calorie diabetic diet

    k. The elderly patient with diabetes is prone to:
       (1) Urinary tract infections
       (2) Foot and leg ulcers
       (3) Pruritus
       (4) Vaginitis
       (5) Recurrent skin infections
       (6) Sexual dysfunction in women
       (7) Chronic impotence in men

    l. Acute complications of diabetes and its therapy are serious problems in the elderly patient, requiring prompt intervention to prevent further morbidity or death; these include:
       (1) Diabetic ketoacidosis
       (2) Hyperglycemic nonketotic hyperosmolar coma
       (3) Hypoglycemia

    m. Long-term complications of diabetes include:
       (1) Vascular disease
       (2) Atherosclerosis
       (3) Diabetic retinopathy
       (4) Peripheral and autonomic neuropathy
       (5) Nephropathy

2. Possible assessment findings

    a. The elderly patient may be asymptomatic

    b. Classic signs and symptoms of elevated blood glucose levels, such as polyuria, polydipsia, polyphagia, and weight loss, may not appear in the elderly patient

    c. Signs and symptoms in the elderly patient may include fatigue, infection, and evidence of neuropathy, such as sensory changes

   d. A sudden weight gain commonly precedes diabetes in the elderly patient
   e. Urine glucose level may not be an accurate indicator of elevated blood glucose in the elderly patient because of an increased threshold for urinary glucose excretion
   f. Laboratory test results include fasting blood sugar level above 140 mg/dl, confirmed by a second test, and oral glucose tolerance test results using age-corrected norms for interpretation of results
3. Possible nursing implications
   a. Keep in mind that the nursing goal is to assist the elderly patient with life-style changes to control diabetes and limit the disease effects on the body
   b. Assist the elderly patient in modifying diet so it meets requirements and satisfies personal preference
   c. Expect to administer insulin or oral hypoglycemic medications
   d. Observe for signs and symptoms of hypoglycemic reaction, such as tremors, diaphoresis, tachycardia, and altered level of consciousness
   e. Teach the patient about:
      (1) Self-testing of blood glucose or urine
      (2) Diet modification
      (3) Insulin administration
      (4) Oral hypoglycemic agents
      (5) Hypoglycemic reactions
      (6) Care during concurrent illness
      (7) Foot care
   f. Evaluate the patient's ability to draw up the correct insulin dosage and administer the injection safely
   g. Provide the patient with a written medication schedule
   h. Assist the patient in planning an individualized exercise program
   i. Instruct the patient to perform mouth care twice daily to prevent fungal infections that may occur under dentures and at the corners of the mouth, common in the diabetic patient
   j. Teach the patient how to perform proper foot care and daily foot inspection; stress its importance
   k. Teach the patient to avoid factors that impair circulation, such as smoking, crossing legs, cold environment, tight-fitting clothing, knee-length hose, furniture that presses against the calf or back of knee
   l. Teach the patient the importance of proper daily skin care; emphasize the need to avoid complications from extreme temperatures, irritation, trauma, and infection
   m. Advise the newly diagnosed diabetic patient to have an ophthalmologic examination
4. Evaluation: base on
   a. Serum glucose levels within normal range for the elderly diabetic patient
   b. Successful adaptation to therapeutic regimen
   c. Proper management of complications of diabetes mellitus

J. Diverticular disease
1. General information
   a. Diverticular disease is the most common colon disease in the Western world
   b. Diverticulosis is a usually asymptomatic disorder in which sac-like herniations of the mucous membrane (diverticula) push through muscle fibers of the intestine
   c. Diverticula usually begin to develop around age 50, increasing in size and number with age
   d. Forty percent of persons over age 70 are estimated to have diverticulosis
   e. Risk factors for diverticulosis include:
      (1) Age
      (2) Obesity
      (3) Constipation
      (4) Hiatal hernia
      (5) History of diet high in refined, low-residue foods
      (6) Emotional tension
   f. A serious complication in the elderly person with diverticulosis is diverticulitis (inflammation of diverticula)
      (1) Obesity, eating irritating foods, drinking alcohol, excessive coughing, or straining while having a bowel movement may precipitate diverticulitis in the patient with diverticulosis
      (2) Possible complications of diverticulitis include intestinal perforation, severe bleeding, peritonitis, abscesses, fistulae, and obstruction
   g. Treatment varies according to the severity of symptoms
   h. The elderly person who does not yet have signs and symptoms of diverticular disease can benefit from measures to prevent its development, such as eating a high-fiber diet and preventing constipation
   i. Careful investigation of gastrointestinal complaints in the elderly person is important to rule out other more serious disorders, such as colon cancer
2. Possible assessment findings
   a. The person with diverticulosis may be asymptomatic
   b. Signs and symptoms of diverticulosis may include:
      (1) Change in bowel habits; usually constipation or diarrhea, or constipation alternating with diarrhea
      (2) Tenderness or pain in the lower left quadrant that increases in severity at a definite time interval after meals or following an emotional disturbance
   c. Signs and symptoms of diverticulitis may range from mild to severe with sudden onset and may include:
      (1) Abdominal pain
      (2) Chills
      (3) Fever
      (4) Nausea
      (5) Rebound tenderness
      (6) Rectal bleeding

      d. Barium enema may reveal spasms in muscles around diverticula; spasms produce narrowing, obstruction, hypermotility, and other changes

      e. Sigmoidoscopy and flexible colonoscopy may reveal irritability and spasm of the colon

  3. Possible nursing implications

      a. Keep in mind that the nursing goal is to relieve signs and symptoms and prevent recurrence and complications of diverticular disease

      b. Remember the following interventions for the patient with acute diverticulitis:

        (1) Promote bed rest

        (2) Give only fluids or withhold food and fluids, as ordered

        (3) Expect to administer I.V. therapy to maintain fluid and electrolyte balance

        (4) Emphasize the importance of progressing from a low-residue to a high-residue diet

        (5) Administer blood replacement, as ordered, in acute diverticulitis with bleeding

        (6) Expect to administer analgesics, sedatives, spasmolytic agents, local heat, and antibiotics

      c. Teach the patient the importance of a high-fiber diet to manage and prevent diverticular disease

      d. Be aware of special problems the elderly patient may have with a high-fiber diet, such as:

        (1) Diet may include more food than patient can reasonably ingest

        (2) Teeth in poor condition or ill-fitting dentures may make eating a high-fiber diet difficult

        (3) Flatulence, distention, and diarrhea may occur

      e. Emphasize the importance of preventing or relieving constipation

      f. Teach measures to prevent constipation, such as:

        (1) Maintaining a high fluid intake to soften stool

        (2) Increasing daily exercise, if possible

      g. Avoid using a bed pan for patient, if possible; instead, assist the elderly patient to the toilet or bedside commode to facilitate proper position and use of abdominal muscles when having a bowel movement

      h. Provide privacy and an unhurried atmosphere while patient uses toilet

  4. Evaluation: base on prevention and relief of signs and symptoms of diverticular disease

K. Fractures

  1. General information

      a. A fracture is a partial or complete disruption in bone continuity

      b. The risk of sustaining a serious fracture increases after age 40

      c. Elderly persons are more susceptible to fractures from even minimal forces because of their high incidence of osteoporosis, osteomalacia, and age-related bone loss

   d. Common chronic conditions, such as arthritis, cataracts, glaucoma, and neurologic problems that affect gait or limit vision or mobility, may result in increased falls and fractures

   e. Fractures should be treated promptly; untreated or inadequately treated fractures can result in permanent disability and dependency

   f. Fractures in younger persons usually occur in the bone shaft; fractures in elderly persons usually occur in cancellous bone near joints

   g. Fractures are more common in elderly women than elderly men

   h. Such age-related changes as weakened muscles, tendons, and cartilage from the loss of elasticity increase the incidence of fractures in elderly persons

   i. The percentage of falls that result in fractures increases with age

   j. The most common fracture sites in elderly persons include:
     (1) Vertebrae
     (2) Upper end of femur (hip fracture)
     (3) Distal end of radius (Colles' fracture)
     (4) Proximal end of humerus

   k. Fractures of the upper end of the femur are the most common and potentially the most disabling

   l. Fractures of the femoral neck carry the greatest risk of nonunion and posttraumatic degenerative joint disease because the blood supply to the femoral head runs through the femoral neck

   m. A hip fracture is the most serious kind of fracture for elderly persons

   n. At highest risk for a hip fracture is the elderly woman living alone

   o. Successful recovery of elderly persons from a fracture depends on avoiding complications, such as:
     (1) Permanent disability
     (2) Joint contractures
     (3) Skin breakdown
     (4) Fat emboli syndrome
     (5) Pulmonary emboli
     (6) Nerve damage

   p. Treatment for a fractured hip may involve such surgical procedures as open or closed internal fixation and total hip replacement

2. Possible assessment findings

   a. Signs and symptoms vary depending on the location, severity, and type of fracture as well as the length of time before seeking treatment

   b. Possible signs and symptoms for all types of fractures include the following:
     (1) Pain
     (2) Inability to move the injured part
     (3) Pallor
     (4) Ecchymosis
     (5) Tenderness localized to a specific point
     (6) Paresthesia
     (7) Edema

(8) Deformity

(9) Crepitus

(10) Confusion

c. Although specific signs and symptoms vary depending on the type of hip fracture, the affected limb will usually show:

(1) Shortening

(2) Flexion

(3) Weakness

(4) External foot rotation

(5) Pain at the knee and/or fracture site (although pain may also be absent)

d. Dehydration, skin breakdown, and hypothermia may occur if an elderly person living alone falls and isn't found for several hours

e. X-rays of the affected area determine the location, extent, and severity of the fracture

f. If the patient has a hip fracture, complete blood count, type and cross-matching, electrolyte levels, and prothrombin and partial thromboplastin times may be ordered

g. Neurovascular assessment of the area distal to the fracture will help determine if vascular or nerve damage has occurred

3. Possible nursing implications

a. Keep in mind that the nursing goal is to facilitate rehabilitation, limit immobility, prevent complications, and prevent other falls

b. Assist with fracture immobilization

c. Perform frequent neurovascular assessments of the area distal to the fracture

d. Provide meticulous care to all exposed skin around the injury

e. Teach the patient proper cast care, if appropriate

f. Assist with an exercise program to prevent immobility

g. Provide patient teaching to prevent future falls

(1) Help patients identify and correct any home safety hazards

(2) Caution against taking medications that cause drowsiness while performing daily activities that would increase the risk of a fall, such as vacuuming

(3) Encourage elderly persons to be alert to environmental hazards that cause falls, such as wet floors or loose carpets

(4) Warn patients not to go outside in icy weather, if possible

(5) Help patients identify behaviors that increase the risk of falls, such as rushing to answer the telephone

(6) Help patients overcome their fear of falling by using these prevention techniques

4. Evaluation: base on

a. Successful recovery without disability from a fracture

b. Successful patient awareness of how to prevent future falls

L. Glaucoma
1. General information
   a. Glaucoma is a group of disorders characterized by increased intraocular pressure, which can damage the optic nerve
   b. Three types of glaucoma usually affect elderly persons:
      (1) Acute glaucoma, a sudden increase in intraocular pressure from a narrowing of the anterior chamber angle
      (2) Chronic open-angle glaucoma, an insidious onset of increased intraocular pressure from a defect in the outflow of aqueous humor
      (3) Chronic closed-angle glaucoma, an insidious onset of increased intraocular pressure from a narrowing of the anterior chamber angle
   c. The lens thickening that occurs with aging can result in a shallow anterior chamber, predisposing the person to glaucoma
   d. Untreated glaucoma can lead to vision loss and blindness
   e. Chronic open-angle glaucoma, the most common type in elderly persons, affects 90% of all patients with glaucoma and exhibits a hereditary tendency
2. Possible assessment findings
   a. Signs and symptoms depend on the type of glaucoma
   b. Chronic open-angle glaucoma is usually bilateral with insidious onset and a slowly progressive course; signs and symptoms appear late in the disease and include:
      (1) Mild aching in the eyes
      (2) Loss of peripheral vision
      (3) Seeing halos around lights
      (4) Reduced visual acuity (especially at night)
      (5) Vague headaches
   c. Chronic closed-angle glaucoma is characterized by intermittent attacks of increased intraocular pressure that resolve spontaneously; signs and symptoms are the same as for chronic open-angle glaucoma
   d. Acute closed-angle glaucoma is unilateral; signs and symptoms are abrupt in onset and include:
      (1) Excruciating pain
      (2) Nausea and vomiting
      (3) Inflammation
      (4) Seeing halos around lights
      (5) Dilated pupil that is nonreactive to light
      (6) Globe is hard to the touch
      (7) Cornea is cloudy
   e. Diagnostic tests include tonometry to measure intraocular pressure, slit-lamp examination of the anterior eye structures and gonioscopy to determine the anterior chamber angle
3. Possible nursing implications
   a. Keep in mind that the nursing goal is to prevent vision loss
   b. Encourage elderly persons to have yearly eye examinations that include intraocular pressure measurement

    c. For chronic open-angle glaucoma, expect to administer eye drops to decrease aqueous humor production, or miotics, such as pilocarpine, to facilitate the outflow of aqueous humor

    d. Remember that chronic glaucoma can be treated with an argon laser trabeculoplasty or trabeculectomy and iridectomy

    e. For acute closed-angle glaucoma, expect to administer timolol maleate (Timoptic Solution), miotic eye drops, intravenous medications (e.g., a carbonic anhydrase inhibitor or hyperosmotic agent to rapidly decrease intraocular pressure by decreasing the formation of aqueous humor), and pain medication; if drugs don't lower the pressure, laser surgery or iridectomy is performed

    f. Teach the patient how to administer eye drops and the side effects of all drugs

    g. Stress the importance of meticulous daily compliance with the prescribed drug therapy to prevent increased intraocular pressure

  4. Evaluation: base on

    a. Successful decrease in intraocular pressure

    b. Successful patient awareness of the importance of drug therapy

M. Hypertension

  1. General information

    a. Hypertension is persistent elevation in diastolic or systolic blood pressure above that considered normal for a given age

    b. Controversy exists over what constitutes normal blood pressure and hypertension in the elderly person

    c. Age-related changes that may contribute to hypertension in the elderly person include:

      (1) Aortic rigidity

      (2) Decreased baroreceptor sensitivity

      (3) Decreased arteriole lumen size

      (4) Reduced glomerular filtration

      (5) Changes in renin-angiotensin system

      (6) Hormonal and cardiovascular changes

    d. Risk factors include:

      (1) Heredity

      (2) Obesity

      (3) Stress

      (4) Diet high in saturated fats or sodium

      (5) Cigarette smoking

      (6) Sedentary life-style

    e. Hypertension is a major risk factor for cardiovascular disease in the elderly person; it predisposes the elderly person to cerebrovascular accidents, cardiac disease, and renal failure

    f. When systolic blood pressure increases with exercise, it takes longer to return to resting levels in the elderly person compared to younger person

    g. Systolic and diastolic blood pressure increase slightly up to age 70 in both men and women

    h. Systolic blood pressure may decline slightly in women over age 70

    i. Systolic pressure may increase more rapidly than diastolic pressure, resulting in a widened pulse pressure

    j. Two types of hypertension occur

      (1) Essential (idiopathic or primary) hypertension: has no identifiable cause and may be multifactorial in origin

      (2) Secondary hypertension: has an underlying cause

    k. Isolated systolic hypertension in the elderly person may result from:

      (1) Severe anemia

      (2) Paget's disease

      (3) Thyrotoxicosis

      (4) Aortic regurgitation

    l. Diastolic hypertension after age 60 may occur if an atherosclerotic lesion in a renal artery develops a thrombosis or embolus

2. Possible assessment findings

    a. Controversy exists about treatment of hypertension in the elderly person

    b. In many cases, diagnosis is based on blood pressure elevations of more than 150/95 mm Hg in person over age 50 taken on three different occasions

    c. Signs and symptoms may include:

      (1) Dull headache on awakening

      (2) Impaired memory

      (3) Nausea and vomiting

      (4) Epistaxis

      (5) Slow tremor

    d. Patient may be asymptomatic

3. Possible nursing implications

    a. Keep in mind that the nursing goal is gradual reduction in the patient's blood pressure to the goal set by the doctor

    b. Take blood pressure readings with patient in at least two different positions, lying or sitting and standing, to detect postural changes

    c. Help the patient reduce dietary sodium through education and meal planning; explain how to read food packaging labels to determine food's sodium content

    d. Promote a restful and stress-free environment; encourage regular exercise

    e. If patient is obese, assist in weight reduction plan

    f. Teach the patient about antihypertensive medications, including how to avoid and cope with a hypotensive reaction:

      (1) Move slowly from sitting or lying position

      (2) Avoid standing motionless, hot baths, and excessive alcohol intake

      (3) Use caution when driving within 2 hours after taking an antihypertensive medication

      (4) If hypotension occurs, lie down with feet elevated to increase cerebral blood flow

g. If thiazide diuretics are ordered, teach patient importance of potassium replacement

h. Remember that adrenergic blocking agents may cause sudden changes in blood pressure because their action is less predictable and more difficult to control in the elderly patient

i. Assess for other side effects of antihypertensive therapy that may mimic stereotypes associated with aging, such as dizziness, impaired vision, and inability to walk properly

4. Evaluation: base on

a. Attainment and maintenance of patient's goal blood pressure

b. Prevention of hypertensive crisis

N. Hypothyroidism

1. General information

a. Hypothyroidism usually occurs after age 50

b. Hypothyroidism is a state of low serum thyroid hormone and its effect on body tissues

c. Possible causes of inadequate production of thyroid hormone include:

(1) Dysfunction of thyroid gland from surgery, irradiation therapy, inflammation, chronic immune thyroiditis (Hashimoto's disease), or such inflammatory conditions as amyloidosis and sarcoidosis

(2) Pituitary failure to produce thyroid-stimulating hormone

(3) Hypothalamic failure to produce thyrotropin-releasing hormone

(4) Iodine deficiency, usually dietary

(5) Antithyroid medications used for thyrotoxicosis

d. Signs and symptoms of hypothyroidism may be similar to normal aging changes, making it difficult to detect hypothyroidism in elderly patients

e. Difficulty of recognizing hypothyroidism in elderly patients is also attributed to its insidious onset

f. Elderly patients may have varying degrees of hypothyroidism

g. Elderly patients with hypothyroidism are at greater risk of developing myxedema coma, a life-threatening and advanced stage of the disease; this usually occurs in those with preexisting, and perhaps undiagnosed, hypothyroidism after such precipitating factors as infections, trauma, and drugs that suppress the central nervous system

h. Hypothyroidism is treated by replacement of thyroid hormone

i. Increased cholesterol levels and a high incidence of atherosclerosis or coronary disease frequently occur in elderly patients with hypothyroidism

j. A weakened cardiac muscle (a normal consequence of aging) makes elderly patients susceptible to coronary insufficiency, congestive heart failure, and cardiac arrest—especially after too vigorous an approach to replacement therapy

2. Possible assessment findings

a. Keep in mind that the clinical signs and symptoms of hypothyroidism in elderly patients may be masked by its similarity to normal aging changes

b. Signs and symptoms of hypothyroidism include:
(1) Change in mental status, such as apathy, forgetfulness, and sleepiness, which may be mistaken for ordinary confusion
(2) Metabolic abnormalities, such as cold intolerance, weakness, lassitude, and low energy
(3) Circulatory impairments, such as decreased cardiac output, heart rate, and blood pressure
(4) Respiratory problems, such as decreased respiratory rate and dyspnea on exertion
(5) Gastrointestinal signs, such as weight gain, constipation, and poor appetite
(6) Sluggish motor activity with hypoactive reflexes
c. The patient's general appearance includes such features as thickened dry skin, sparse dry hair, brittle nails, and anemia. Easy bruising and nonpitting edema characterized by putty face, hands, and feet may also be evident
d. Radioimmunoassay indicates low T3 and T4 levels
e. Thyroid-stimulating hormone levels may be increased in hypothyroidism because of thyroid insufficiency or decreased because of hypothalamic or pituitary insufficiency
f. Elevated levels of serum cholesterol, carotene, alkaline phosphatase, and triglycerides may be present
g. Normocytic normochromic anemia may be present
h. Laboratory tests in myxedema coma may indicate low serum sodium and arterial blood gases may show decreased pH and increased PCO_2, indicating respiratory acidosis from a decreased respiratory rate
i. Signs and symptoms of myxedema coma include:
(1) Hypothermia
(2) Hypoventilation
(3) Hypotension
(4) Hypoactive reflexes
(5) Bradycardia
(6) Cool, dry skin
(7) Seizures
(8) Edema in the face (especially the periorbital region) and extremities
(9) Decreased level of consciousness, ranging from slow mentation to stupor and coma
3. Possible nursing implications
a. Keep in mind that the nursing goal is to provide support and comfort while restoring euthyroidism
b. Nursing interventions during myxedema coma are as follows:
(1) Monitor temperature, intake and output, vital signs, arterial blood gases, and serum electrolyte levels
(2) Provide skin care and turn the bedridden patient with edema at least every 2 hours

(3) Maintain a patent I.V. line

(4) Avoid sedation, if possible, or reduce dosage

(5) Provide oxygen or possibly mechanical ventilation for respiratory assistance

(6) Expect to administer thyroid hormone intravenously

   c. Remember that an unduly aggressive treatment of hypothyroidism can cause adverse cardiac effects, such as chest pain or tachycardia

   d. Watch for hypertension and congestive heart failure in elderly patients receiving thyroid hormone replacement

   e. Infections may precipitate myxedema coma; check for possible infectious sources, such as in blood, urine, and sputum

   f. Teach the patient/family the importance of continued treatment and medical supervision

   g. Caution the patient that abrupt withdrawal from replacement therapy can precipitate myxedema coma

   h. Assess the patient for signs of hyperthyroidism during replacement therapy

   i. Instruct the patient to promptly report chest pain and tachycardia

   j. Teach the patient the importance of promptly seeking medical attention for infections

   k. Provide a warm environment and adequate clothing during replacement therapy

   l. Consider the patient's limitations when planning activities

   m. Promote good nutrition and prevent constipation by providing a high-protein, low-calorie, high-fiber diet

   n. Apply lotion to dry skin when needed

  4. Evaluation: base on

   a. Successful restoration and maintenance of euthyroidism

   b. Successful patient/family teaching that includes the following:

(1) Signs and symptoms of medication overdose

(2) Hazards of noncompliance

(3) Understanding the necessity of lifetime replacement therapy

O. Arterial insufficiency

  1. General information

   a. Arterial insufficiency may result from:

(1) Arterial embolism

(2) Arterial thrombosis

(3) Arteriosclerosis obliterans

(4) Vascular changes in diabetes mellitus

(5) Trauma

   b. Risk factors include:

(1) Male sex with an inherited predisposition to cardiovascular disease or peripheral vascular disease and a history of hypertension

(2) Smoking

(3) Diabetes mellitus

(4) Hypercholesterolemia

(5) Obesity

(6) Stressful life-style

c. Arteriosclerosis obliterans is the most frequent cause of arterial disease resulting in ischemic lesions of the extremities in elderly patients

d. Clinical manifestations of arteriosclerosis obliterans and its management depend on the location and extent of the occlusive process

e. The femoral, popliteal, and tibial arteries are most frequently involved in elderly patients; the aorta and iliac artery may also be involved

f. Peripheral arterial disease in the patient with diabetes mellitus is complicated by three major etiologic factors:

(1) Occlusive arterial disease

(2) Neuropathy

(3) Infection

g. Diabetes mellitus has been found to accelerate the process by which arteriosclerosis obliterans develops

h. Patients at high risk for developing acute arterial occlusion include:

(1) Those who have undergone arterial invasive procedures, such as an arteriogram

(2) Those with atrial fibrillation

(3) Those recovering from vascular surgery

(4) Those with a proximal aneurysm of the abdominal aorta or popliteal artery

(5) Those with lacerated, severed, or compressed arteries

2. Possible assessment findings

a. Pain may be sudden in acute arterial insufficiency or gradual in chronic arterial insufficiency

b. Intermittent claudication may be present and relieved by rest in chronic arterial insufficiency

c. Pulses in the affected extremity may be absent or weak

d. The patient with chronic arterial insufficiency may exhibit the following changes in the legs and feet:

(1) Thin, dry, and shiny skin

(2) Thickened nails

(3) Absence of hair

(4) Possible temperature variations

(5) Pallor on elevation

(6) Dependent erythema

(7) Atrophy with a decrease in limb size

e. Ulcers may be present between the toes or at the tip of the toes, over phalangeal heads, on the heel, over the lateral malleolus or pretibial area, and in the diabetic patient, over the metatarsal heads and on the side or sole of the foot

f. Ulcer characteristics in chronic arterial insufficiency include:

(1) Well-defined edges

(2) Black or necrotic tissue

(3) Deep base and pale in color

(4) Absence of bleeding

g. The patient with acute arterial occlusion will have a sudden onset of symptoms indicating a complete arterial blockage, which can cause serious tissue ischemia

h. Signs and symptoms of acute arterial occlusion include:

(1) Sudden burning or aching pain in an area distal to the occlusion

(2) Pain aggravated with movement

(3) Numbness

(4) Pallor

(5) Coldness

(6) Weakness

(7) Paresthesia

(8) Weak or absent pulse

(9) Occlusion site will be tender to touch

i. Treatment for acute arterial occlusion depends on the cause of the occlusion and the patient's general health

3. Possible nursing implications

a. Keep in mind that the nursing goal is to identify early signs of acute and chronic arterial insufficiency in order to forestall ischemic changes and relieve pain in affected extremities

b. Chronic arterial insufficiency

(1) Encourage the patient to engage in a progressive walking program to promote the development of collateral circulation

(2) Recommend that the patient take slow walks two or three times a day, taking short steps, avoiding stairs and hills, and gradually increasing the distance

(3) Advise the patient to stop when pain is present

(4) If the patient has a history of angina, exercise must be modified to prevent anginal pain

(5) Teach the elderly person with arterial insufficiency how to control such associated risk factors as obesity, smoking, diabetes, or hypercholesteremia

(6) Administer analgesics or narcotics for pain relief

(7) Teach the patient the importance of meticulous daily foot care in preventing ischemic ulcers and infection

(8) Suggest the patient place lamb's wool between overlapping toes to separate them and prevent ulceration

(9) Advise the patient to avoid extremes of hot and cold; heating pads, hot water bottles, and hot soaks should not be used

(10) Advise the patient to avoid constricting garments, such as girdles, garters, and tight hose or shoes

c. Acute arterial insufficiency

(1) Protect the affected limb by keeping it straight and at room temperature

(2) Expect to administer anticoagulation therapy

(3) Frequently assess pulses and motor and sensory responses in the affected limb

(4) Check for symmetry in the size and shape of limbs

4. Evaluation: base on
   a. Successful management of symptoms and improved arterial circulation
   b. Prevention of ischemic changes

P. Venous insufficiency

1. General information
   a. Age-related vascular changes have been associated with the development of varicosity, thrombophlebitis, and chronic venous insufficiency from valvular destruction
   b. Varicose veins usually affect the superficial veins, such as the greater and lesser saphenous veins
   c. Varicose veins result from structural changes in the venous walls and valves, resulting in the pooling of blood and edema; the veins become increasingly dilated, tortuous, and serpentine in appearance
   d. Elderly patients with varicose veins are at high risk of developing venous thrombosis
   e. The increased incidence of venous thrombosis in elderly patients has been associated with a progressive enlargement of the intramuscular calf veins, which occurs with aging
   f. Precipitating factors related to venous thrombophlebitis include:
      (1) Any stress that injures the intima of vessels
      (2) Altered blood coagulability
      (3) Blood stasis
      (4) Fractures
      (5) Immobility
      (6) Surgery
      (7) Obesity
      (8) Debilitating diseases, such as congestive heart failure, neoplasms, chronic infections, or stroke
   g. Deep venous thrombosis involves veins in the calf, including the peroneal and posterior tibial veins
   h. Superficial venous thrombosis usually involves the greater and lesser saphenous veins and is usually self-limiting
   i. Deep venous thrombosis is a serious condition placing the patient at risk for pulmonary embolism
   j. Bed rest places the elderly patient at increased risk for venous thrombosis
   k. Venous thrombosis rarely develops without associated inflammation; in thrombophlebitis, both a thrombus and inflammation are present
   l. Signs and symptoms of thrombophlebitis include:
      (1) Tenderness, redness, and warmth over a hard stringlike vein
      (2) Homans' sign (calf pain with dorsiflexion of the foot)
      (3) Edema in the affected extremity

    m. Chronic venous insufficiency will produce:
      (1) Chronic leg edema
      (2) Tissue fibrosis and induration
      (3) Skin discoloration from extravasation of blood in subcutaneous tissue
      (4) Stasis ulcers

2. Possible assessment findings
    a. Varicose veins may appear swollen, distended, and knotted and are usually located in the subcutaneous tissues of the legs
    b. Varicose veins develop gradually and may be asymptomatic or may exhibit mild to severe symptoms
    c. Signs and symptoms of varicose veins may include:
      (1) A feeling of leg heaviness
      (2) Leg cramps at night
      (3) Diffuse, dull aching pain after standing or walking
      (4) Fatigability
      (5) Palpable nodules
    d. In advanced stages, varicose veins may become thick and hard to the touch with dull or stabbing pain; impaired circulation may cause ulcers in the lower legs
    e. Diagnostic tests to detect venous thrombosis include:
      (1) Contrast venography
      (2) Doppler ultrasonography
      (3) Radioactive-labeled fibrinogen
      (4) Impedance plethysmography
      (5) Phlebography

3. Possible nursing implications
    a. Keep in mind that the nursing goal is to promote comfort and minimize varicosities and to prevent the formation of thrombi or emboli
    b. Advise the patient with varicose veins against wearing constrictive clothing
    c. Suggest antiembolism stockings to promote venous return; stockings should be worn from the proximal foot to just below the knee and should be applied after the leg has been elevated for 5 minutes to prevent blood trapping
    d. Encourage the patient to elevate his legs periodically during the day for 1 to 2 hours
    e. Advise the patient to avoid prolonged standing
    f. Encourage regular walking to prevent venous stasis
    g. Teach the patient to be alert for the development of thrombophlebitis and stasis ulcers
    h. Be familiar with the nursing implications of specific medications and surgical treatments
    i. Remember that nursing care for thrombophlebitis may include:
      (1) Bed rest for 4 to 10 days, as prescribed
      (2) Leg elevation to decrease pain, edema, and venous stasis

      (3) Elastic stockings that may be used while in bed and should always be used when ambulating to compress the veins and promote venous return

      (4) Avoidance of prolonged sitting or standing

      (5) Application of warm moist packs to the entire length of the extremity to relieve vasospasm and inflammation

      (6) Administration of anticoagulation therapy, or fibrinolytic medication

  j. Be alert for signs and symptoms of pulmonary emboli, such as dyspnea, chest pain, and tachycardia; if pulmonary embolism is suspected, promptly notify the doctor

4. Evaluation: base on
   a. Successive management and relief of symptoms
   b. Assessment for and prevention of complications
   c. Prevention of stasis ulcers

Q. Myocardial infarction (MI)

1. General information
   a. MI occurs when blood flow through one or more of the coronary arteries is obstructed and results in severe myocardial ischemia and necrosis
   b. Mortality rate from MI is twice as high for persons over age 70 as it is for younger persons
   c. Age-related changes in blood, vessel walls, and hemodynamics increase the risk of MI in the elderly person
   d. Physical exertion or eating a large meal may precipitate an MI in a susceptible elderly person
   e. MI occurs in men and women at approximately equal rates
   f. Risk factors for MI include:
      (1) Family history
      (2) Hypertension
      (3) Obesity
      (4) Diabetes mellitus
      (5) Smoking
      (6) Stress
      (7) Sedentary life-style
      (8) High serum cholesterol and/or triglyceride levels
   g. Silent MI (no apparent signs and symptoms) commonly occurs in elderly persons and in many cases results in sudden death
   h. The elderly MI patient is at risk of developing such complications as:
      (1) Serious dysrhythmias
      (2) Congestive heart failure
      (3) Cardiogenic shock
      (4) Digitalis toxicity with digitalis therapy
      (5) Cardiac rupture
2. Possible assessment findings
   a. Signs and symptoms commonly are subtle and variable; the elderly person may develop:
      (1) Dyspnea

(2) Sudden mental deterioration

(3) Dizziness

(4) Intense and prolonged weakness and fatigue

(5) Feeling of faintness

(6) Loss of consciousness

(7) Abdominal distress

(8) Vomiting

(9) Hiccups

(10) Palpitations

b. Pain or other signs and symptoms may be absent in the elderly person

c. MI in the elderly person may result in progressive renal failure with uremia; embolic occlusion of noncerebral arteries with ischemia or peripheral gangrene may also occur

d. EKG may show elevated ST segment and inverted T waves; EKG changes are difficult to interpret because of possible preexisting cardiac disease

e. Laboratory test results include elevated SGOT, LDH, and CPK levels

3. Possible nursing implications

a. Keep in mind that the nursing goal is to decrease cardiac work load

b. Assess pain and administer analgesics; monitor for side effects

c. Expect to administer sedatives

d. Be aware that sedatives may produce psychosis and sensory deprivation in the elderly patient, especially while in a coronary care unit; sedatives may also result in feeding difficulty, increasing the risk of aspiration pneumonia

e. Assist and monitor exercise; chair rest for short periods is preferable to bed rest

f. Observe for signs and symptoms of systemic emboli, pulmonary emboli, and venous thrombosis

g. Expect to administer anticoagulants; carefully assess for any bleeding

h. Provide psychosocial support and education regarding MI and rehabilitation

i. Teach patient importance of progressive cardiac rehabilitation

j. Confirm that patient understands prescribed activity plan, medications, and the importance of follow-up medical care

4. Evaluation: base on successful recovery and adaptation to any life-style changes as a result of MI

R. Osteoarthritis

1. General information

a. Osteoarthritis is a nonsystemic joint disease that mainly affects elderly persons

b. Osteoarthritis is characterized by a breakdown of articular cartilage with bone hypertrophy at the margins and synovial membrane changes

c. Areas most affected by osteoarthritis include:

(1) Hip joint

        (2) Knee
        (3) Distal interphalangeal joints
        (4) Proximal interphalangeal joints
        (5) Cervical spine
        (6) Lumbosacral spine

    d. Osteoarthritis may be classified as primary (idiopathic) or secondary (caused by other conditions)

    e. Factors that influence the progression of osteoarthritis include aging, trauma, obesity, heredity, prior inflammatory disease, and metabolic and endocrine disorders

    f. Osteoarthritis usually progresses slowly

    g. Discomfort and stiffness may increasingly immobilize elderly patients and disrupt or restrict their day-to-day activities and life-style

2. Possible assessment findings

    a. Symptoms vary from mild to severe depending on the amount of joint degeneration

    b. Aching joint pain and stiffness usually increases after overuse or inactivity

    c. Pain and stiffness after activity is often relieved by rest

    d. Stiffness upon awakening or after inactivity usually improves with exercise or activity

    e. Loss of joint mobility and stiffness may make even simple movements painful

    f. Posture and gait abnormalities may be caused by muscle weakness

    g. Crepitus (a crunching or grating sound) may be heard when roughened articular or extra-articular surfaces come in contact with each other

    h. X-ray examination usually reveals narrowing of the joint space, bony changes, and spur formation

    i. Spurs called Heberden's nodes may develop at distal interphalangeal finger joints; Bouchard's nodes may be present on the proximal interphalangeal finger joints

3. Possible nursing implications

    a. Keep in mind that the nursing goal is to relieve discomfort, maintain range of motion, and prevent crippling deformities

    b. If aspirin is used, be alert for side effects, such as tinnitus, gastrointestinal upset, and occult blood loss

    c. If nonsteroidal anti-inflammatory agents are used, counsel the patient about side effects, such as gastrointestinal upset

    d. Physical therapy including heat, ultrasound, and massage may relieve discomfort of cervical and lumbosacral osteoarthritis

    e. Hip and knee replacements may relieve symptoms and restore independence in elderly patients

    f. Assist with planning weight reduction programs, if recommended

    g. Apply traction or a cervical collar to relieve nerve root pressure in the neck, if appropriate

    h. Encourage daily exercise to maintain maximum range of motion

      i. Encourage the use of walkers or canes to reduce strain on weight-bearing joints, if necessary

  4. Evaluation: base on the successful management of pain and maintenance of maximum joint mobility

S. Osteoporosis

  1. General information

    a. Osteoporosis is a bone disorder in which an imbalance between bone formation and resorption results in bone demineralization

    b. Bone demineralization results in bones that become porous, brittle, and abnormally vulnerable to fracture

    c. Some osteoporosis is a normal aging change

    d. Some 15 to 20 million Americans have osteoporosis

    e. Factors associated with osteoporosis include:

      (1) Normal aging

      (2) Hereditary factors

      (3) Small constitutional size

      (4) Inactivity

      (5) Estrogen deficiency in postmenopausal women

      (6) Calcium deficiency

      (7) Nutritional status

      (8) Prolonged corticosteroid administration

      (9) Prolonged heparin therapy

     (10) Alcoholism

     (11) Diabetes mellitus

     (12) Cigarette smoking

     (13) Rheumatoid arthritis

    f. Fractures resulting from osteoporosis pose a serious threat to the elderly person's independence

    g. In advanced osteoporosis, vertebral compression fractures and kyphosis can compress heart, lungs, and nerves and decrease thorax mobility; this can cause respiratory and cardiac difficulties

    h. U.S. health care costs related to osteoporosis are estimated at $3 million

    i. Women have rapid bone loss for 5 years after menopause

    j. Osteoporosis is eight times more common in women than men

    k. The ability to absorb calcium from the intestines decreases with age, which may contribute to osteoporosis

  2. Possible assessment findings

    a. Osteoporosis may develop insidiously

    b. Complaints may be vague, such as easy fatigability, general weakness in the limbs, headache, and a feeling of insecurity when walking

    c. The person's height may decrease over months or years

    d. Compression fractures of the vertebrae, especially lower thoracic and lumbar, produce a lower dorsal kyphosis ("dowager's hump" or "widow's hump") with abdominal protrusion

    e. Ribs and the iliac crest angle downward

    f. The rounded back and the shortened trunk may make the extremities appear disproportionately long

    g. Changes in respiratory function may result from the decreased size of the thorax

    h. Bending and stair-climbing may be difficult because of limited movement

    i. Fractures, especially in the wrist (Colles' fracture), vertebrae (T12, L1), and hip, may occur from only minor trauma

    j. Diagnostic tests are performed to rule out conditions, such as osteoarthritis, that may masquerade as osteoporosis

    k. Serum calcium, inorganic phosphorus, and alkaline phosphatase levels are normal in the elderly person with osteoporosis

    l. Serum alkaline phosphatase levels usually rise moderately after a fracture and remain elevated for several weeks

    m. X-rays may show degeneration in the lower thoracic and lumbar vertebrae

    n. Bone biopsy reveals thin, porous, but otherwise normal bone

3. Possible nursing implications

    a. Keep in mind that the nursing goal is to slow or halt bone loss, remineralize bone, and minimize danger of falls

    b. Teach the patient ways to carry out daily activities without sudden bending or lifting or carrying heavy objects

    c. Teach patient safety precautions to avoid falls, such as using nonskid rugs to prevent slipping, wearing well-fitting low-heel shoes, installing clear lighting, and keeping pathways unobstructed

    d. Advise patient to follow high-calcium diet with adequate fluoride and vitamin D; warn against excessive phosphorus intake

    e. Administer analgesics for pain

    f. If estrogen therapy is ordered, advise the patient of side effects; emphasize the importance of close follow-up and ongoing reevaluation

    g. Encourage the patient to engage in an exercise program carefully planned to match condition and capability; this tends to strengthen bones

    h. Provide psychological support to the patient with osteoporosis who is coping with alterations in body image and life-style

4. Evaluation: base on minimizing bone loss and preventing fractures

T. Renal failure

1. General information

    a. Renal failure is the inability of the kidney to excrete body metabolites; it may be acute or chronic

    b. Chronic renal failure has increased among the elderly population

    c. Urinary tract infections and renovascular disease from hypertension are the leading causes of renal impairment in elderly persons

    d. Normal aging changes in renal function place the elderly person at a higher risk of developing renal failure from any compromise in renal function

    e. Renal failure in the elderly person may result if the following conditions are left untreated or treatment is delayed or inadequate:
       (1) Inadequate fluid intake
       (2) Fluid loss from diarrhea, vomiting, or hemorrhage
       (3) Cardiac failure
       (4) Inappropriate use of diuretics and laxatives
       (5) Urinary tract infections
       (6) Urinary tract obstruction caused by calculi or prostatic hypertrophy

    f. Causes of acute renal failure in the elderly person include:
       (1) Hypotensive episode
       (2) Antibiotic overdose
       (3) Hypovolemia

    g. Acute renal failure can develop into chronic renal failure in the elderly person

    h. Chronic renal failure in the elderly person commonly results from other chronic illnesses, such as uncontrolled hypertension and diabetes mellitus; other causes include chronic glomerulonephritis, polycystic kidney disease, and cancer

    i. The prognosis for the patient with renal failure depends on the presence of other organic or systemic diseases and the patient's ability to adapt to disease, therapy, and life-style changes

    j. Common complications of renal failure in the elderly person include:
       (1) Anemia
       (2) Renal osteodystrophy
       (3) Hypertension
       (4) Dysrhythmias
       (5) Congestive heart failure
       (6) Pericarditis
       (7) Central and peripheral nervous system neuropathy
       (8) Dry, itchy skin

    k. Renal failure affects every body system

    l. The elderly person with chronic renal failure usually has three treatment options, including:
       (1) Conservative treatment: goal is preservation of remaining function, treatment of any reversible causes of renal failure, and relief of symptoms caused by uremia
       (2) Hemodialysis: waste products and excess water are removed by circulating blood through a dialyzer
       (3) Peritoneal dialysis: cleansing fluid is instilled into peritoneal cavity to remove waste products and fluid through osmosis

2. Possible assessment findings
    a. Early assessment of renal failure may be difficult, because normal aging changes and other disease processes may mask signs and symptoms
    b. Initially, hyponatremia may occur, producing hypotension, dry mouth, loss of skin turgor, listlessness, fatigue, and nausea; later, somnolence (sleepiness) and confusion may develop; as disease process further

progresses, sodium retention, hyperkalemia, and fluid overload may occur

c. As urine output decreases, urine may become dilute and contain casts and crystals

d. Hypertension may occur from fluid or sodium excess or excess renin production

e. Congestive heart failure may develop from fluid overload

f. Uremia may cause inflammation of pericardium

g. Dysrhythmias may develop from electrolyte imbalance

h. Dyspnea and pulmonary congestion may develop because of congestive heart failure

i. Kussmaul's respirations may result from acidosis

j. Person with renal failure has increased susceptibility to infection
(1) This may result in staphylococcal infections of dialysis shunts, fistulae, peritoneal catheters, and open wounds
(2) *Candida albicans*, a common bacteria affecting the buccal mucosa, causes formation of white plaques that may develop into ulcers that can spread to the esophagus and result in dysphagia

k. Dry mouth, metallic taste, and uremic odor may be present

l. Anorexia, nausea, and vomiting may occur

m. Inflammation and ulcerations may occur along the gastrointestinal tract

n. Anemia may occur; the degree varies as do its signs and symptoms

o. Bleeding and clotting disorders occur in late renal failure with the following clinical manifestations:
(1) Epistaxis
(2) Increased occult intestinal blood loss
(3) Bruising after trauma

p. Neuropathy occurs from the buildup of uremic waste products; characterized by tingling and restlessness usually in the lower extremities and loss of motor strength and grip

q. Headache, lassitude, memory changes, and decrease in mental function may occur

r. Skin may have a yellow or sallow tone

s. Bone demineralization may occur
(1) Early in the disease process the patient may be asymptomatic
(2) Later, bone pain and stress fractures may occur, and deposits of calcium phosphate crystals may develop in soft tissues of muscles, joints, and blood vessels

t. Blood urea nitrogen level is elevated (greater than 70 mg/dl)

u. Creatinine level is elevated using age-corrected norms

v. Uric acid and serum phosphorus levels may be elevated; serum calcium levels may be low

w. Urinalysis may show protein, glucose, erythrocytes, leukocytes, and casts

x. Urine specific gravity may be fixed at 1.010

y. Kidney biopsy may be performed to determine underlying pathology

3. Possible nursing implications
   a. Keep in mind that the nursing goal is symptomatic relief, prevention of complications, and assistance to patient in maintaining an acceptable quality of life
   b. Instruct the patient about adhering to a diet low in protein, potassium, and sodium by careful meal planning
   c. Teach the patient the importance of following prescribed fluid restriction
   d. Teach the patient the importance of frequent and meticulous mouth care to prevent oral infections
   e. Monitor for signs and symptoms of hyperkalemia:
      (1) Cramping of legs and abdomen
      (2) Diarrhea
   f. Monitor for signs and symptoms of fluid overload:
      (1) Edema
      (2) Weight gain
      (3) Hypertension
      (4) Shortness of breath
      (5) Orthopnea
      (6) Crackles
   g. Explain the importance of skin care, using superfatted soaps, oatmeal baths, and skin lotion to manage pruritus
   h. Help the anemic patient cope with low energy levels by restructuring activities and setting priorities for energy expenditure
   i. Help the elderly patient follow the multiple-medication regimen by giving careful instruction, reinforcing instruction, and developing reminders to simplify the task
   j. Monitor for side effects, interactions, and complications of medications
   k. Monitor for joint or bone complications; reinforce the importance of safety measures to prevent fractures
   l. Be familiar with specific nursing implications regarding hemodialysis and peritoneal dialysis
   m. Foster independence by encouraging the patient to take part in decision making and to maximize activity
   n. Provide support and understanding to the patient and family
   o. Support the patient and family in decision making about continuing treatment when dialysis is poorly tolerated and the patient becomes dependent or mentally incapacitated
   p. Provide emotional and physical comfort to the patient who terminates treatment
4. Evaluation: base on
   a. Successful management of symptoms
   b. Successful adaptation to life-style changes related to diet, medication, activity level, and dialysis treatments

U. Thyrotoxicosis
1. General information
   a. Thyrotoxicosis is a disorder caused by excessive thyroid hormone production and its effect on body tissues
   b. Disorders most frequently associated with thyrotoxicosis include:
      (1) Graves' disease
      (2) Toxic nodular goiters
      (3) Subacute thyroiditis
   c. Signs and symptoms of thyrotoxicosis may be absent or attributed to other more common diseases in elderly persons
   d. The cause of thyrotoxicosis is unknown; autoimmune, psychological, traumatic, and hereditary factors have been implicated
   e. Primary forms of treatment include:
      (1) Antithyroid drugs
      (2) ^{131}I
      (3) Surgery
   f. Thyrotoxicosis in an elderly patient may precipitate congestive heart failure, acute pulmonary edema, and angina
2. Possible assessment findings
   a. Symptoms of thyrotoxicosis may include:
      (1) Nervousness and/or tremor
      (2) Weight loss
      (3) Heat intolerance with excessive perspiration
      (4) Emotional lability
      (5) Proximal muscle weakness
      (6) Diarrhea
      (7) Tachycardia
      (8) Widened pulse pressure
      (9) Warm, smooth skin
      (10) Thyroid enlargement or abnormality
      (11) Exophthalmos, although less common in elderly patients
   b. Signs and symptoms of thyrotoxicosis may not be clearly evident in elderly patients
   c. Weight loss and congestive heart failure may be the predominant symptoms of thyrotoxicosis in elderly patients
   d. Other common symptoms in elderly patients include:
      (1) Continuous nervousness
      (2) Fine tremors
      (3) Weight loss despite excellent appetite
      (4) Tachycardia that does not disappear during sleep or after rest
   e. Thyrotoxic crisis (thyroid storm) is an acute manifestation of thyrotoxicosis, usually occurring in patients with preexisting (though frequently unrecognized) disease; its onset is abrupt and precipitated by a stressful event (such as trauma, surgery, or infection) and can be fatal if untreated

    f. Elevated serum protein-bound iodine reflects increased thyroid activity

    g. Radioimmunoassay indicates increased serum T4 and T3 concentrations

    h. Thyrotropin-releasing hormone stimulation test indicates the failure of thyroid-stimulating hormone levels to increase within 30 minutes after the administration of thyrotropin-releasing hormone

3. Possible nursing implications

    a. Keep in mind that the nursing goal is to restore the patient to euthyroidism and provide support and comfort during thyrotoxicosis

    b. Monitor:

        (1) Vital signs

        (2) Level of consciousness

        (3) Serum electrolytes

        (4) Cardiac function

        (5) Urinary output

    c. Emphasize the importance of bed rest

    d. Provide a quiet, dark, and comfortable environment to facilitate rest and minimize stimuli

    e. Be familiar with nursing implications specific to the patient's therapeutic regimen

    f. Be alert for signs of thyrotoxic crisis, such as tachycardia, irritability, hyperkinesia, high fever, visual disturbances, vomiting, diarrhea, and hypertension

    g. Provide eye care to the patient with exophthalmos or ophthalmopathy by moistening conjunctivae with isotonic eye drops and suggesting that eyeglasses or eye patches be worn to protect the eyes

    h. Instruct the patient about the importance of a high-calorie, nutritious diet with vitamin supplements

    i. Expect to administer sedatives to promote rest

    j. Counsel the patient and family about the course of the disease and to expect that the patient may be emotionally labile at times

    k. Emphasize the importance of a quiet, nonstimulating environment

    l. Stress the importance of regular medical follow-up

4. Evaluation: base on successful restoration and maintenance of euthyroidism without complications

V. Urinary tract infection (UTI)

1. General information

    a. UTI incidence increases with age

    b. Debilitated and chronically ill patients are at high risk for developing UTI and possible severe complications

    c. UTI occurs more commonly in women, because of their shorter urethra, than in men

    d. Elderly men are more at risk than younger men for developing UTI because of prostatic hypertrophy

    e. UTI is usually caused by *Escherichia coli* or other gram-negative enteric bacteria

    f. Risk factors for UTI include:
- (1) Urinary stasis, retention, and obstruction
- (2) Institutionalization, which increases exposure to bacteria
- (3) Diabetes mellitus
- (4) Renal failure
- (5) Hypertension
- (6) Cerebrovascular accident (CVA)
- (7) Dementia
- (8) Sexual activity
- (9) Use of catheters and other instrumentation

    g. Conditions that predispose elderly patients to urinary stasis, retention, and obstruction include:
- (1) Urethral or ureteral stenosis
- (2) Urethral or ureteral strictures
- (3) Renal calculi
- (4) Immobility
- (5) Tumors
- (6) Neurologic changes from CVAs
- (7) Cystocele in women
- (8) Prostatic hypertrophy in men

    h. If untreated, UTI may progress to bacteremia or renal failure

    i. The decision to treat asymptomatic bacteriuria in elderly patients varies among doctors

2. Possible assessment findings

    a. The elderly patient with UTI may be asymptomatic or exhibit vague, ill-defined symptoms

    b. Symptoms may include:
- (1) Lower abdominal discomfort
- (2) Urinary frequency
- (3) Urinary urgency
- (4) Dysuria
- (5) Nocturia
- (6) Turbid urine
- (7) Fever
- (8) Chills
- (9) Hematuria
- (10) Vomiting

    c. Quantitative urine culture revealing a bacterial count of 100,000/ml or more confirms diagnosis

    d. Gram stain identifies bacteria type

    e. A follow-up culture is performed after 10 days to determine effectiveness of antibiotic therapy

3. Possible nursing implications

    a. Keep in mind that the nursing goal is to resolve and prevent UTI

    b. Explain the importance of maintaining adequate fluid intake (2,500 to 3,000 ml in 24 hours)

    c. Verify urine cultures, organism, drug sensitivity, and drug allergies before initiating antibiotic therapy

    d. Emphasize the importance of strict compliance with antibiotic therapy regimen; teach about possible side effects

    e. Write out schedule for antibiotic therapy with specific instructions; e.g., take 1 hour before or after meals

    f. Teach the sexually active elderly person to prevent UTI by such methods as voiding immediately after intercourse, bathing before and after intercourse, and using alternative positions to decrease stress placed on the woman's urethra by the male superior position

    g. Teach the elderly person proper perineal hygiene (cleansing perineum from front to back) to prevent fecal bacteria from entering the urethra

    h. Advise the elderly person prone to UTI of possible benefits of a diet that promotes acid urine to prevent growth of pathogens; such foods include prunes, plums, cranberries, grains, meats, eggs, cheese, and fish

    i. Promote periodic activity and meticulous perineal care for patient with limited mobility

    j. Suspect and investigate for possible UTI when patient's voiding habits change

    k. Teach the patient the purpose of medications used to prevent or decrease frequency of UTI, such as methenamine salts (Mandelamine, Hiprex) and nitrofurantoin (Furadantin and Macrodantin)

    l. Instruct the patient to avoid such irritating chemicals as harsh soaps, powders, bubble baths, and deodorants when cleansing the perineal area because they can change perineum pH and impair tissue integrity

    m. Caution the patient against ingesting caffeine, which may irritate the bladder

    n. Recommend warm sitz baths to help relieve discomfort

    o. Warn the patient that his urine may turn red-orange if phenazopyridine, a urinary analgesic, is ordered.

    p. Advise the patient to urinate at the first urge

    q. Suggest that women wear pantyhose with a ventilated cotton crotch and cotton, rather than synthetic-fiber, underpants to allow ventilation of the perineum and absorption of vaginal discharge

    r. Follow proper aseptic technique during Foley catheter insertion

    s. Maintain a sterile closed system when using a urinary drainage system; keep in mind the major entry points for bacteria: the urethral meatus, the junction between the catheter and the collection tube, the connection to the drainage bag, and the open end of the drainage spigot

    t. Position drainage bag below bladder level and off the floor

    u. Teach both patient and family the principles of proper Foley catheter maintenance

4. Evaluation: base on

    a. Resolution of UTI

    b. Prevention of UTI

    c. Proper management of Foley catheter

Points to Remember

Signs and symptoms of several pathologic health problems in elderly persons may be subtle and variable and are often different from those seen in younger persons.

Cataracts are one of the most common eye problems affecting elderly persons.

Chronic obstructive pulmonary disease is the major cause of respiratory disability in elderly patients.

Immobility is the single biggest risk factor for developing decubitus ulcers.

The two most common types of dementia are multi-infarct dementia and Alzheimer's disease.

Glucose intolerance among elderly persons may occur from aging changes in insulin levels, insulin release, peripheral effectiveness of insulin, or a combination of these.

Normal aging changes place elderly persons at a higher risk of developing renal failure from any compromise in renal function.

Glossary

Exacerbation—an increase in the severity of a disease or in the intensity of any of its signs or symptoms

Hemianopia—loss of vision in half the visual field (usually the vertical half) of one or both eyes

Hyperkinesis—abnormally increased motor activity

Miotic—an agent that constricts pupils

Proprioception—the sensation of body position, movement, and equilibrium changes from specialized nerve endings located mainly in muscles, tendons, and the labyrinth of the inner ear

Pulse pressure—the numerical difference between systolic blood pressure and diastolic blood pressure; normally 30 to 40 mm Hg

Stenosis—a narrowing or constriction of an opening or passageway

Valsalva's maneuver—forced expiration effort against a closed glottis, such as when a person holds his breath and tenses his muscles to change position in bed; the resultant increased intrathoracic pressure decreases venous blood return to the right side of the heart

Functional Health Problems

Learning Objectives

After studying this section, the reader should be able to:

• Describe a functional assessment.

• Define sensory deprivation.

• Identify assessment findings that indicate impaired function in each of the following areas: auditory function, visual function, taste and smell, and integumentary function.

• Identify assessment findings associated with impaired mobility.

• Describe assessment findings associated with urinary incontinence.

• State two nursing interventions for each of the following functional problems: sensory deprivation, auditory impairment, visual impairment, taste and smell alteration, impaired integumentary function, impaired mobility, and urinary incontinence.

VI. Functional Health Problems

A. Functional assessment

1. General information
   a. Functional assessment is a method that nurses can use to measure the older adult's overall well-being and self-care abilities
   b. Functional assessment can identify individual needs and care deficits
   c. Assessment findings provide the basis for developing a care plan that preserves and enhances the older adult's abilities in the presence of coexisting disease and chronic illness
   d. Functional assessment can identify and match such services as housekeeping, home health care, day care, etc., with the older adult's needs to maintain his independence
   e. Functional assessment can provide feedback regarding treatment and rehabilitation
   f. Functional assessment tools must be evaluated for reliability and validity

2. Types of functional assessment
   a. Assessment of Activities of Daily Living: measures ability to perform daily personal care, such as feeding, bathing, toileting, and dressing
   b. Assessment of Instrumental Activities of Daily Living: assesses the ability to perform more complex personal-care activities, such as cooking, cleaning, and shopping

3. Functional assessment tools
   a. PULSES (Physical condition, Upper limbs, Lower limbs, Social factors, Sensory component) Profile: measures level of independence and dependence in performing activities of daily living
   b. Barthel Index and Barthel Self-Care Rating: measures physical dependence in performing personal care
   c. FANCAPES (Fluid, Aeration, Nutrition, Communication, Activity, Pain, Elimination, Socialization): evaluates ability to meet needs and the extent to which assistance is necessary
   d. OARS (Older Adult Resource Services) Multidimensional Functional Assessment: evaluates ability, disability, and the capability level at which the person can function; it assesses the following functional capabilities: social resources, economic resources, physical health, mental health, and activities of daily living

B. Sensory deprivation

1. General information
   a. Sensory deprivation is characterized by:
      (1) Decrease in sensory input
      (2) Decrease in meaningful activity or relevance of stimuli
      (3) Alteration in the reticular activating system
   b. Sensory impairments in the elderly person are cumulative, occur over time, compound each other, and can result in or potentiate sensory deprivation

c. Sensory deprivation, distortion, and overload may coexist for the elderly person
d. Factors that make the elderly person particularly vulnerable to misperception or decreased perception of sensory stimuli include:
(1) Physiologic changes associated with aging or illness that interfere with perception or reception of stimuli
(2) Structural characteristics of the environment or treatment forms that either distort, disrupt, monotonize, mute, intensify, or disorganize stimuli in such a way that they eliminate the order and meaning of stimuli
(3) Caregiver expectations of appropriate behavior; behaviors that would facilitate interpretation of stimuli, such as exploring and verbally communicating, may be discouraged or prohibited by nursing staff and others
e. Acute health problems, such as dehydration, high fever, and shock may cause sensory alteration in the elderly person, making him vulnerable to sensory deprivation
f. Social isolation is a major component of sensory deprivation for the elderly person
g. Sensory deprivation may be mislabeled or overlooked because manifestations of sensory deprivation in the elderly person are similar to those associated with what people consider to be senility
2. Possible assessment findings
a. Responses to sensory deprivation vary from individual to individual
b. Changes in cognitive function because of sensory deprivation may include:
(1) Confusion
(2) Disorientation
(3) General slowing of intellectual activity
(4) Difficulty in concentration, abstract thinking, and ability to think coherently and solve problems
c. Emotional responses may include:
(1) Anxiety
(2) Fear
(3) Depression
(4) Rapid mood swings
d. Perceptual changes from sensory deprivation may be visual, auditory, kinesthetic, or somasthetic, varying from mild daydreams to illusions and hallucinations
e. Behavioral changes may include noncompliant behavior, wandering, and purposeless activity
3. Possible nursing implications
a. Keep in mind that the nursing goal is to promote the optimal level of sensory input
b. Be aware that sensory deprivation results from a combination of physiologic, psychological, and environmental factors

    c. Maximize remaining sensory function to help decrease sensory deprivation by correcting deficits, such as helping the elderly person get eyeglasses and hearing aids

    d. Use touch to help orient the elderly person and provide stimulation

    e. Provide all the cues the person needs to maintain orientation and sense of reality, such as clocks, calendars, and a predictable daily routine

    f. Encourage the person to participate in activities within his ability

    g. Provide various activities and inputs

    h. Be aware that background entertainment, such as television or radio, may turn into background noise and disturbance

    i. Allow the elderly person control over stimulation level

    j. Allow the person to gain knowledge and awareness of the environment through exploring, handling and touching, asking questions, and verbalizing

    k. Provide opportunities for problem solving and independent decision making; make every attempt to make problem solving successful and meaningful

    l. Facilitate interaction between the elderly person and others in his environment

    m. Provide goal-directed, focused conversations on topics meaningful to him

C. Auditory impairment

  1. General information

    a. Auditory impairment is the most problematic sensory loss

    b. Sound distortion affects interpretation of the world, which can lead to social isolation, depression, paranoia, suspiciousness, and impaired problem-solving ability because the affected person cannot hear information

    c. 30% of persons over age 65 have hearing loss, 13% need professional assistance, twice as many men as women have hearing loss

    d. Auditory changes occur subtly over time

    e. Presbycusis is a progressive, bilaterally symmetrical sensorineural hearing loss that occurs with age

    f. Sensorineural hearing loss is a dysfunction in transmission of sound to the brain

    g. Conductive hearing loss results from an impediment in the mechanical transmission of sound along the auditory pathway; may improve with medical treatment or hearing aids

    h. Mixed hearing loss refers to the presence of both conductive and sensorineural losses

    i. Presbycusis affects the ability to hear high-pitched sounds and sibilant consonants such as f, s, th, ch, and sh. As hearing loss progresses, perception of the consonants b, t, p, k, and d is also impaired

    j. Clear perception of consonants is important in understanding language with high-pitched sounds

    k. Excessive cerumen in the middle ear will intensify presbycusis

l. Background noise can further impair the hearing ability of the elderly person with presbycusis

2. Possible assessment findings

   a. Detection of hearing loss may be difficult because of the person's adaptation to hearing loss over time

   b. Subtle cues of hearing loss include inappropriate response to questions or failure to respond to questions

   c. The elderly person with impaired hearing may have difficulty following verbal directions

   d. The elderly person with impaired hearing may withdraw from social conversation

   e. The person may frequently ask for clarification and repetition

   f. The person may turn one ear to the speaker while watching the speaker intently

   g. The person's speech may have an unusual quality with poor articulation; it may be too loud or too soft, monotonous or harsh

   h. The elderly person with conductive hearing loss experiences a loss of hearing sensitivity that is usually the same for all frequencies; speech discrimination may be unimpaired if speech is loud enough

   i. The elderly person with sensorineural hearing loss has difficulty understanding speech even when it is loud enough to be heard

3. Possible nursing implications

   a. Keep in mind that the nursing goal is to maximize auditory function

   b. Determine extent of loss by audiologic examination; complete assessment and evaluation are essential to determine appropriate treatment

   c. Modify communication skills to help the hearing-impaired person:
      (1) Face the person
      (2) Get his attention by touch or eye contact
      (3) Sit or stand so he can see your lips
      (4) Speak slowly and distinctly
      (5) Speak in voice loud enough to be heard without shouting
      (6) Use short phrases
      (7) Use body language
      (8) Eliminate as much background noise as possible
      (9) Use speaking tubes or hearing horns for the severely hearing-impaired person if necessary

   d. Motivate the person to try a hearing aid, needed by many older adults; the type of aid must be individualized to address the person's needs and type of hearing loss

   e. Tell the person that he will need time to adjust to wearing the hearing aid and to learn to use and care for the equipment; he will need to change compensatory patterns already established, such as asking people to repeat or not paying attention to conversational cues, to decrease social isolation

   f. Suggest auditory aids to foster independence, including amplifiers on telephone receivers, telephone bell amplifiers, lighted signals on

telephones, and auxiliary speakers for radios, televisions, and tape recorders
- g. Note at main nursing station intercom that patient is deaf or hearing impaired
- h. When teaching the hearing-impaired person, ask him to repeat learning points to ensure that content was heard
- i. Be aware that the hearing-impaired older person is often ignored or assumed to be senile; nursing has a major advocacy role to play in promoting assessment and evaluation for auditory impairment

D. Visual impairment
1. General information
   - a. Presbyopia, a condition that occurs with aging, is a decrease in the ability of the eye to accommodate, usually resulting in hyperopia (farsightedness)
   - b. Physiologic changes in the eye from aging produce decreased accommodation, senile miosis, increased lens opacity, decreased peripheral vision, and lens yellowing
   - c. Rhodopsin (visual purple) breakdown in response to light rays decreases, contributing to poor adaptation to darkness
   - d. Macular degeneration is a condition in the elderly person caused by hardening and obstruction of retinal arteries; it results in loss of central vision while peripheral vision remains unimpaired
   - e. Diabetic retinopathy is a condition in which microaneurysms and small hemorrhages occur in or on the retina, resulting in vision loss
   - f. Glaucoma, a condition characterized by increased intraocular pressure, can result in damage to the optic nerve and, possibly, blindness; onset of glaucoma may be acute or gradual (see "Glaucoma," page 73)
   - g. Cataract is the development of opacity of the lens of the eye (see "Cataracts," page 52)
   - h. Visual loss in the elderly person increases susceptibility to illusions, withdrawal, disorientation, and interpersonal isolation
2. Possible assessment findings
   - a. With decreased accommodation, the visually impaired person may hold objects at a distance to focus properly on them
   - b. The elderly person may have difficulty with color perception of blues, violets, and greens
   - c. Vision may be impaired in dim light
   - d. Panoramic vision may be impaired
   - e. Tonometry examination in the patient with glaucoma reveals increased intraocular pressure
   - f. The elderly person with glaucoma may complain of eyestrain and morning headaches that disappear after rising
   - g. The elderly person with cataracts may complain of poor vision, eye fatigue, headaches, increased light sensitivity, and blurred vision or multiple images

      h. The elderly person with macular degeneration may complain that his central vision is dark or distorted

  3. Possible nursing implications

      a. Keep in mind that the nursing goal is to maximize visual function

      b. Help the visually impaired person develop compensatory skills

      c. Help the person with macular degeneration to maximize use of peripheral vision

      d. Support the postsurgery cataract patient in adjusting to distorted vision and eyeglasses or contact lenses

      e. Be aware that rehabilitation plans should maximize use of nonvisual aids

      f. Suggest visual aids to foster independence, including:

        (1) Large-print books and magazines

        (2) Recorded books

        (3) Magnifying glass

        (4) Plastic-page device that magnifies a printed page

        (5) Lighted mirror

        (6) Large-number push-button telephone

      g. Be aware that associations for the blind and other community programs can assist with travel, talking books

      h. Assess ability to meet ADLs; assist with environmental changes needed to facilitate independent living

      i. Provide support to the elderly person who has recently experienced blindness or vision impairment that alters self-image, self-esteem, and confidence to function independently

E. Alterations in taste and smell

  1. General information

      a. The number of taste buds per papilla decreases with age

      b. Taste buds that distinguish sweet and salty flavors show the greatest decline with age

      c. Loss of taste and smell has direct effects on dietary intake and food enjoyment

      d. Ability to taste is associated with ability to smell

      e. Smoking and mouth condition affect ability to taste

      f. Ability to smell begins to decline at age 45

      g. With decline of smell, older adults may not detect smoke

  2. Possible assessment findings

      a. The elderly person may heavily season food with salt or strong spices to compensate for taste alterations

      b. The elderly person may add extra sugar to coffee or tea

      c. The elderly person may prefer very sweet or salty foods

  3. Possible nursing implications

      a. Keep in mind that the nursing goal is to maximize taste and smell function

      b. Educate the elderly person about aging changes in taste and smell

      c. Find substitutes for salt and sugar such as spices and seasoning, as indicated by the elderly person's medical history

    d. Do not assume the elderly person needs a bland diet

    e. Encourage use of smoke detectors to alert the elderly person of a fire

F. Impaired integument
1. General information
    a. Generalized thinning of skin occurs with aging
    b. Dry skin in the elderly person results from decreased sebaceous gland activity, thinning of the epidermal layer, and poor fluid intake
    c. The elderly person is more prone to skin dryness from environmental elements, decreased humidity, use of harsh soap, frequent bathing, and nutritional deficiencies
    d. Itching (pruritus) from skin dryness threatens skin integrity
    e. Other causes of itching, such as scabies, pediculosis, and intertrigo, should be ruled out
    f. Skin turgor decreases with age, resulting in stiffer, less pliable skin
    g. Wound healing is slower in the elderly person
2. Possible assessment findings
    a. Rough, scaly, flaking skin may appear on the face, neck, hands, forearms, sides of the lower trunk, and the exterior and lateral aspects of the thighs
    b. Itching may accompany dryness; skin irritation or scratch marks may be present
    c. Dryness and itching are generally aggravated by cold, dry, wintry weather, exposure to sun and wind, and irritating fabrics or wool
    d. Skin may bruise easily; hemorrhages, known as senile purpura, may be present
3. Possible nursing implications
    a. Keep in mind that the nursing goal is to maintain integumentary function and prevent skin breakdown
    b. Use superfatted soaps to restore protective lipid film to skin surface
    c. Incorporate bath oils and other hydrophobic preparations into bathing routine
    d. Apply lotions or emollients to the body to help lubricate and hydrate epidermal layer
    e. Maintain adequate humidity in environment
    f. Advise the elderly person to avoid irritating clothing and hot baths and showers and to limit the number of showers and baths
    g. Advise the elderly person to maintain adequate fluid intake

G. Impaired mobility
1. General information
    a. Decreased mobility is a serious problem for the elderly person
    b. Conditions that commonly limit mobility include paresthesias, arthritis, neuromotor disturbances, fractures, energy-depleting illnesses, stroke, joint or foot pain, angina, and peripheral vascular disease

    c. Movement capabilities can be maintained into old age by continuous use

    d. Foot problems have a tremendous impact on immobility

    e. Complications associated with bed rest and lack of physical mobility include:

      (1) Muscle atrophy

      (2) Contractures

      (3) Osteoporosis

      (4) Decubitus ulcers

      (5) Orthostatic hypotension

      (6) Urinary calculi

      (7) Dehydration

      (8) Thromboemboli and pulmonary emboli

      (9) Poor appetite

     (10) Constipation

     (11) Fatigue

     (12) Insomnia

     (13) Stress

     (14) Depression

    f. Gait disturbances may develop in the elderly person

    g. Impaired mobility increases risk of injury and falls

2. Possible assessment findings

    a. The elderly person may limit mobility because of poor eyesight or joint and foot discomfort

    b. The elderly person may limit mobility because of fear of falling

    c. Gait disturbances may be present

    d. Lack of well-fitting shoes and assistive devices, such as canes and walkers, may restrict mobility

    e. Mobility and activity level may be limited because of low energy level or depression

    f. Immobility may occur after hospitalization or confinement to bed because of illness

3. Possible nursing interventions

    a. Keep in mind that the nursing goal is to maximize mobility and prevent falls

    b. Suggest ambulatory aids to foster independence: walkers, including wheeled walkers and those with seats; canes, including tripod canes; wheelchairs, including motorized wheelchairs; Canadian crutches; lifter chairs

    c. Encourage the elderly person to engage in a systematic exercise program, tailored to individual capabilities, that has been approved by his doctor

    d. Educate the elderly person about the benefits of exercise and activity

    e. Assist and encourage the elderly person who is confined to a wheelchair or bed to engage in a modified exercise program

    f. Perform passive range-of-motion exercises for the elderly bedridden patient to prevent contractures and to keep joints straight

g. Assist the elderly bedridden patient in performing active exercise to prevent muscle atrophy

h. Avoid flexion postures when positioning the elderly bedridden patient to prevent knee and hip contractures

i. Ensure that the elderly patient who is confined to chair or wheelchair receives range-of-motion exercises to prevent knee and hip contractures that can result from sitting all day

j. Teach the elderly person the importance of foot care and well-fitting shoes

k. Support and encourage the elderly patient receiving physical therapy following a hip fracture or prolonged bed rest

l. Teach safety measures specific to individual needs to prevent injury and falls

H. Urinary incontinence

1. General information
   a. Urinary incontinence is the inability to control loss of urine
   b. Types of incontinence include:

      (1) Stress incontinence: incompetent bladder outlet caused by weakness of supporting pelvic muscles; mainly affects women; incontinence occurs when a woman sneezes, coughs, or laughs

      (2) Overflow incontinence: overflow caused by obstructive lesion or drug-induced retention; associated with obstructive problems in women, prostate problems in men

      (3) Neurogenic incontinence: alteration in sensory and motor tracts involved in bladder muscle function

      (4) Urgency incontinence: sudden urge to void followed by loss of large amounts of urine

   c. Urinary incontinence affects self-esteem, confidence, and independence
   d. Urinary incontinence may produce dependence, shame, guilt, and fear
   e. Incontinence may result from problems that affect toileting, such as generalized weakness or problem with walking to reach bathroom, manipulation of clothing, handling the bedpan or urinal

2. Possible assessment findings
   a. The elderly woman may experience stress incontinence: small amounts of urine are released when she coughs, sneezes, or laughs
   b. The elderly person may experience dribbling from overflow
   c. The elderly person may experience an urge to void followed by incontinence
   d. Urinalysis may reveal infection as a cause of incontinence
   e. A cystometrogram can determine patterns of the bladder's emptying mechanism
   f. A cystogram tests motor and sensory ability of the bladder
   g. Neurologic tests can determine bladder sensation

h. The elderly person taking sleeping medications or tranquilizers may experience incontinence at night because these drugs depress the neurologic sensation that signals the need to urinate

i. Urinary incontinence may occur in the elderly person taking diuretics

j. The elderly person taking medications that cause urinary retention may experience overflow incontinence

3. Possible nursing implications

a. Keep in mind that the nursing goal is to assist with efforts to improve urinary continence

b. Provide frequent opportunities to void if assistance with toileting is needed

c. Modify environment to facilitate toileting: may need to relocate furniture or bedroom and use portable facilities, grab rails in bathroom, or an elevated toilet seat

d. Use Velcro fasteners to replace cumbersome buttons and hooks on clothing

e. Administer estrogen treatment for atrophic vaginitis or urethritis, if ordered

f. Administer antibiotics for acute urinary tract infection, if ordered

g. Assist the elderly person in planning daily activities and ways to manage incontinence

h. Initiate scheduled toileting or bladder retraining to avoid episodes of incontinence

   (1) Provide privacy and warmth
   (2) Toilet patient every 2 hours during day
   (3) Toilet patient every 4 hours during night
   (4) Carefully time fluid intake and medications
   (5) Progressively lengthen or shorten toileting intervals

i. If patient has difficulty voiding, teach techniques to trigger voiding, such as running water, stroking inner thigh, and suprapubic tapping

j. Be aware that indwelling catheters are indicated in the patient with severe urinary retention that causes recurrent, symptomatic urinary tract infection or hydronephrosis and in the patient with skin rashes, ulcers, and wounds that are irritated by contact with urine

k. Teach Kegel exercises to elderly woman with stress incontinence to strengthen pelvic floor muscles

   (1) Instruct the woman to identify muscles of pelvic floor by placing finger inside vagina or rectum and squeezing around finger; these are the same muscles used to hold back gas or a bowel movement
   (2) Instruct woman not to contract stomach, leg, or buttock muscles
   (3) Tell her to squeeze identified muscle for 10 seconds and relax for 10 seconds
   (4) Instruct her to do 15 exercises in the morning, 15 in the afternoon, and 20 at night or to do exercise for 10 minutes three times a day
   (5) Tell her to work up to 25 exercises at a time
   (6) Explain that she will notice change in 2 weeks to 1 month if exercises are consistently done on a daily basis

Points to Remember

Functional assessment tools may be helpful in matching services with the elderly person's needs to maintain his independence in the community.

Sensory deprivation affects all aspects of life, including functioning and health.

One of the major causes of sensory deprivation is hearing impairment.

Many complications resulting from impaired mobility and lack of physical activity can be prevented in the elderly person.

Incontinence contributes to isolation and loneliness.

Glossary

Functional assessment—assessment that specifically measures self-care ability

Functional assessment tool—an instrument designed to measure self-care ability

Kegel exercise—exercise to strengthen perineal muscles

Stress incontinence—involuntary discharge of urine with increased abdominal pressure from coughing, laughing

Urinary incontinence—inability to control urine excretion

Health Promotion, Safety, and Special Concerns

Learning Objectives

After studying this section, the reader should be able to:

- Cite major physiologic changes from aging that place elderly persons at risk for injury.

- State three major contributing factors of medication problems in elderly persons.

- Cite special precautions for elderly persons engaging in exercise.

- Name three contributing factors to sleep disturbance.

- Identify three common problems with sexual function that older adults experience.

- State three factors that influence diet and nutrition in elderly persons.

VII. Health Promotion, Safety, and Special Concerns

A. Falls
1. General information
   a. Falls rank as the second leading cause of all accidental deaths; about 75% involve older adults
   b. The risk of accidents and complications increases with age
   c. A higher incidence of falls occurs among institutionalized elderly persons
   d. Falls contribute to increased hospital stays and increased costs
   e. In institutions, most falls occur during the evening and night shifts and at change of shifts
   f. Many falls result from environmental hazards
   g. Most falls occur at home
   h. A complex integration of movement, gravity, and equilibrium is necessary for mobility, which may become more difficult with age
   i. Injuries from falls pose a great threat to the well-being of elderly persons, especially those who suffer repeated falls
   j. Women in the old-old age group living alone are at the highest risk for falls
   k. The immobilization necessary after a fall increases the risk of complications in elderly persons
   l. Falls frequently result in hip and wrist fractures in elderly persons
2. Contributing factors
   a. The combination of a weakened skeleton, weakened support system, and changes in the center of gravity predisposes elderly persons to falls and other accidents
   b. Sudden loss of muscle tone without specific cause or loss of consciousness without warning (sometimes referred to as "drop attack") can result in falls
   c. Physical factors contributing to falls include:
      (1) Muscle weakness
      (2) Gait change
      (3) Decreased sensory awareness
      (4) Visual impairment
   d. Environmental factors include:
      (1) Improper footwear
      (2) Obstacles
      (3) Wet floors
      (4) Poor lighting
   e. Cardiovascular disease that results in decreased cardiac output and/or cerebral blood flow increases the risk of falls
   f. Neurologic disorders that result in decreased cerebral blood flow, diminished sensorium, and/or impairment in locomotion also increase the potential of falling
   g. Urinary urgency because of age-related physiologic changes, such as benign prostatic hypertrophy, place the elderly person at risk of falling when rushing to the bathroom

      h. Use of such medications as diuretics (resulting in frequent urination), or hypnotics, tranquilizers, sedatives, and pain medications (all of which can cause drowsiness), have been associated with falls

      i. An increased incidence of falls has been associated with patients using multiple medications and those with multiple medical problems

      j. Altered mental states, such as stress, depression, confusion, and impaired judgment, can contribute to falls and injury

      k. Osteoporosis, which weakens bones, increases the risk of fractures from falls

  3. Possible nursing implications

      a. Keep in mind that the nursing goal is to provide appropriate care for specific fractures and other injuries and to teach elderly persons how to avoid falls

      b. Assess environmental hazards, such as broken stairs, uneven or icy walks, inadequate lighting, frayed carpets, throw rugs, and exposed electric cords

      c. Identify elderly persons at high risk because of advanced age, confusion, unfamiliar surroundings, chronic illnesses, medications that cause sensory impairment, and balance or gait changes

      d. Advise elderly persons to paint the edges of stairs a bright color to increase visibility

      e. Make sure handrails are present and secured

      f. Secure or remove loose carpets and throw rugs

      g. Advise elderly persons to keep outdoor steps and walkways in good repair

      h. Advise elderly persons to use extra caution when going outside during inclement weather

      i. Recommend handrails in bathrooms and nonskid tracks in bathtubs

      j. Advise elderly persons to avoid climbing ladders or using step stools and chairs to reach objects

      k. Advise elderly persons to avoid highly polished floors

      l. Recommend the use of night-lights

      m. Teach elderly persons to change positions slowly to avoid orthostatic hypotension

      n. Encourage elderly persons to wear shoes with adequate support and nonskid heels

B. Hypothermia

  1. General information

      a. Hypothermia is a condition of below-normal body temperature: 95° F. (35° C.) or below

      b. Accidental hypothermia can occur in elderly persons even after exposure to relatively mild cold conditions

      c. Elderly persons at risk include those who have inadequate housing and/or heating, those living alone, those with a chronic illness, and those who have a disorder or are taking a drug that affects the blood vessels' ability to constrict or dilate in response to temperature changes

    d. Preexisiting physical conditions may worsen because hypothermia depresses body functions

    e. Signs and symptoms include the following:

       (1) Skin may appear pale and waxy

       (2) Skin may be cold to touch, but person is not shivering

       (3) Dysrhythmias and bradycardia may be present

       (4) Hypotension may be present

       (5) Muscle rigidity, slurred speech, and drowsiness may occur

2. Contributing factors

    a. Substances that accelerate the loss of body heat, such as alcohol, imipramine, and salicylates, increase the risk of developing hypothermia

    b. Phenothiazines may impair thermoregulation in elderly persons

    c. Elderly patients undergoing surgery are at high risk for developing hypothermia because of:

       (1) Impaired heat regulation from preoperative medications

       (2) Cold operating rooms

       (3) Cold solutions

       (4) Lack of covering

    d. Elderly persons may feel comfortably warm although their bodies are cold; as a result, they may not be aware of lower body temperature and may not take proper precautions to prevent hypothermia

    e. Hypoproteinemia has been associated with hypothermia, which places undernourished elderly persons at risk

3. Possible nursing implications

    a. Keep in mind that the nursing goal is slow rewarming and teaching the patient how to prevent hypothermia

    b. Warm the patient's hands and feet and add covers if hypothermia is suspected

    c. If the core temperature drops below 90° F. (32.2° C.), rewarm the patient slowly under close observation and monitor for cardiac dysrhythmias and hypokalemia

    d. Do not raise body temperature more than 1° F. (0.6° C.) per hour; using electric blankets or hot water bottles can cause vasodilation, resulting in hypotension from an inability to maintain cardiac output

    e. Take the patient's temperature rectally to assess his core body temperature

    f. Keep rooms between 68° F. and 70° F. to prevent hypothermia

    g. Advise elderly persons to dress warmly, eat well, and stay as active as possible

    h. Advise elderly persons to wear enough clothing and use sufficient blankets to keep warm during sleep

    i. Caution elderly persons about drugs that may affect body temperature

    j. If elderly persons live alone, suggest that friends or neighbors call or visit them once or twice a day, especially during cold weather

C. Hyperthermia

1. General information
   a. Hyperthermia has not been specifically defined for the elderly person but is generally considered to be a core body temperature of 100° F. (37.8° C.) or higher
   b. Common causes of hyperthermia in elderly persons include:
      (1) Infection
      (2) An ambient temperature above the body's own temperature
   c. Signs and symptoms vary with the degree of hyperthermia
   d. With a temperature of 100° F., the individual may have apathy, weakness, faintness, and headache; as core body temperature rises, tachycardia, weakness, dry mouth, increased respirations, hallucinations, delusions, and confusion may be present
   e. Heat stroke is characterized by severe tachycardia, severe tachypnea, severe frank hypotension, alteration in consciousness, and a rectal temperature of 105° F. (40.5° C.) or higher
   f. Persons who aren't acclimated to hot weather may suffer from heat syncope, characterized by dizziness, fatigue, and sudden faintness after physical exertion
   g. Heat exhaustion, which is less severe than heat stroke but common in elderly persons, is characterized by orthostatic hypotension, malaise, irritability, anxiety, tachypnea, tachycardia, moderately increased temperature (usually not above 100° F. [37.8° C.]), headache, dizziness, and syncope
   h. Although signs and symptoms overlap, elevated levels of serum glutamic oxaloacetic transaminase (SGOT), lactate dehydrogenase (LDH), and creatinine phosphokinase (CPK) as well as central nervous system disturbances may help distinguish heat stroke from heat exhaustion
2. Contributing factors
   a. A decreased number of sweat glands in elderly persons impairs the body's ability to cool itself
   b. Factors that increase the risk of hyperthermia in elderly persons include:
      (1) Urinary tract infections
      (2) Circulatory problems
      (3) Dehydration
   c. Elderly persons may not be aware of higher body temperatures and, as a result, may not take preventive measures, such as dressing appropriately or using air conditioning and fans
   d. Heat waves have a severe effect on infants and elderly persons
3. Possible nursing implications
   a. Keep in mind that the nursing goal is to reduce body temperature, find the source of hyperthermia, and give supportive care during hyperthermic episodes
   b. For patients with slight hyperthermia, administer cool drinks, reduce clothing to a minimum, reduce activity, sponge face and hands with tepid water, and reduce ambient temperature

    c. For patients with more severe hyperthermia (body temperatures above 103° F. [39.4° C.]), undress the patient and cover his body with sheets or towels wetted with ice chips and water, apply ice packs to the head and back of neck, sponge with tepid water, and then direct dry air over the patient to facilitate cooling

    d. Check rectal temperature frequently during all cooling measures to prevent too rapid a temperature change, which can affect blood pressure and pulse

    e. If the patient begins to shiver, immediately stop the cooling process; shivering will raise body temperature to the previous level

    f. Suspect infection if ambient temperature is below 80° F. (26.6° C.); observe for signs of urinary tract and respiratory infections

    g. Listen and offer comfort to the patient recovering from hyperthermia who has experienced hallucinations or delusions

    h. Prevent hyperthermia by preventing infections, promoting hydration, and teaching elderly persons how to protect themselves from high ambient temperatures

    i. Advise elderly persons during high ambient temperatures to avoid direct sunlight, wear lightweight clothing, use fans, drink cool beverages, eat light, get adequate rest, and avoid physical exertion

D. High altitudes

1. General information

    a. Elderly persons living at high elevations are most unlikely to experience altitude-related illnesses because they have become acclimated

    b. High altitudes may cause hypotensive changes in elderly persons who are not acclimated

    c. High-altitude pulmonary edema, a serious altitude-related illness, includes such signs and symptoms as increasingly severe dyspnea, tachycardia, persistent cough, noisy gurgling respirations, weakness, orthopnea, hemoptysis, and rhonchi and crackles

    d. High-altitude cerebral edema, another serious altitude-related illness, includes such signs and symptoms as increasingly severe headaches, confusion, emotional lability, hallucinations, ataxia, and weakness

2. Contributing factors

    a. Elderly persons with cardiac or respiratory problems may not be able to tolerate a high altitude, even if they are acclimated to it

    b. Strenuous physical exercise at a high altitude may cause unusual or unfamiliar symptoms in anyone, particularly older adults

3. Possible nursing implications

    a. Keep in mind that the goal of nursing care is to prevent altitude-related illness

    b. Advise elderly persons with cardiac and respiratory problems to take special precautions if traveling at high elevations

    c. To care for altitude illness, provide supplemental oxygen and remove the person to a lower elevation

    d. Caution elderly persons living at high altitudes to avoid strenuous physical exercise

E. Fires and burns

  1. General information

    a. Burns can be very disabling to elderly persons because of their slower healing time

    b. Smoke inhalation is particularly deadly in elderly persons who have respiratory disorders or decreased vital capacity

    c. Advanced planning and ongoing training of staff and residents on fire-emergency procedures are necessary in institutional settings where a high risk of accidental fire exists

    d. Fear of fire and of being trapped because of mobility problems are serious concerns to elderly persons

  2. Contributing factors

    a. Decreased sense of smell in elderly persons impairs the ability to detect smoke and gas

    b. Elderly persons may overload old circuitry in their homes or lack the visual acuity to detect frayed electrical cords on lamps and appliances

    c. Decreased sensitivity to heat and pain in elderly persons predispose them to accidental burns

    d. Smoking in bed is a frequent cause of fires

  3. Possible nursing implications

    a. Keep in mind that the nursing goal is to prevent fires and burns

    b. Encourage the use of smoke alarms and regular battery checks

    c. Warn elderly persons of the hazards of extra heating devices, kerosene stoves, gas or electric heaters, and exposed steam pipes

    d. Advise elderly persons not to wear loose-fitting clothing when cooking

    e. Advise elderly persons to make sure heating pads, hot water bottles, and electric blankets are well covered to prevent burns and to use these devices with extreme caution

    f. Advise elderly persons to adjust water heater thermostats so that water from the faucet won't scald them

F. Medication use

  1. General information

    a. Elderly persons are more susceptible to drug-induced illness and adverse effects than younger adults

    b. Sedatives, hypoglycemics, cardiac drugs, and diuretics are the most common drugs prescribed to elderly persons

    c. The four pharmacokinetic processes are absorption, distribution, metabolism, and excretion; all except metabolism are altered in elderly persons

   d. Drug absorption is altered in elderly persons
      (1) Oral drug absorption may be impaired because of mucosal atrophy, decreased gastric emptying, decreased splanchnic blood flow, duodenal diverticula, and decreased motility of the gastrointestinal tract
      (2) Decreased gastric secretion and higher pH may affect the ionization and absorption of some oral drugs
      (3) Intramuscular and subcutaneous drug absorption may be delayed in elderly persons because of reduced blood flow and altered permeability of capillary walls
   e. Drug distribution is altered in elderly persons
      (1) Decreased body weight and total body water lead to higher plasma concentrations of water-soluble drugs
      (2) A decrease in lean body mass along with increased body fat increases the concentration of lipid-soluble drugs, which accumulate in fat and prolong the drug action
      (3) Circulating plasma albumin declines with age, decreasing the number of protein-binding sites for drugs; consequently, the levels of unbound pharmacologically active drugs increase, and this increases the risk of adverse effects and toxicity
   f. No conclusive evidence supporting altered drug metabolism in the elderly person exists
   g. Drug excretion is altered in the elderly person
      (1) Most drugs are eliminated or excreted through the kidneys
      (2) Impaired renal function from aging causes inefficient and slowed drug excretion
      (3) Dehydration, congestive heart failure, pneumonia, urinary tract infection, and renal disease further impair drug excretion
   h. Drugs frequently misused by the elderly person include sleeping pills, antianxiety drugs, pain medications, and laxatives
2. Contributing factors
   a. Response to drug therapy is based on such individual variables as body mass; developmental, physiologic, and psychological states; and drug history
   b. Elderly patients often have multiple pathologic conditions that require multiple medications, increasing the risk of adverse effects
   c. Polypharmacy often exists in the elderly patient because of several factors, including:
      (1) Several medications taken for multiple conditions
      (2) Prescriptions obtained from different doctors
      (3) Over-the-counter drugs used without informing doctors
      (4) Drugs often shared among neighbors and friends
   d. The incidence of drug interactions increases with age and the number of drugs prescribed
   e. Acute and chronic illness may further alter pharmacokinetics in elderly persons

    f. Drug omission is common among elderly persons; contributing factors include:

       (1) Complicated drug therapy schedules

       (2) Memory deficits

       (3) Insufficient income to purchase drugs, unpleasant side effects, and fear that drugs may be habit-forming

    g. Adverse effects, such as confusion, forgetfulness, weakness, or anorexia, may not be recognized because they are mistaken for normal aging changes

3. Possible nursing implications

    a. Keep in mind that the nursing goal is to assist the older adult with responsible medication use

    b. Obtain a complete medical history, including over-the-counter drugs

    c. Verify the patient's ability to read

    d. Monitor the patient's response to drugs and observe for adverse side effects

    e. Monitor plasma concentration of drugs, such as digoxin, antiarrhythmics, antidepressants, and theophylline

    f. Advocate that doctors review prescriptions every 6 months; have the patient take a list of all current medications to doctor visits

    g. Have the patient or a family member show you what and how all medications are taken; e.g., taking over-the-counter laxatives at bedtime with prescribed medications may be inappropriate because of increased bowel transit time

    h. Encourage the person to always use the same pharmacy

    i. Recognize patients at high risk for adverse reactions; risk factors include:

       (1) Multiple chronic illnesses

       (2) Renal failure

       (3) Frail health

       (4) Small build

       (5) Female sex

       (6) History of previous reactions

       (7) History of allergies

       (8) Use of several doctors

       (9) Living alone

      (10) Altered mental state

      (11) Financial difficulty

    j. Teach patients and families:

       (1) To maintain a list of all medications

       (2) How to recognize adverse effects of all prescribed drugs

       (3) To report any drug side effect

       (4) To recognize drug limitations, and help them set realistic expectations

       (5) To place capsules on the front of the tongue and tablets on the back of the tongue for ease of swallowing

       (6) To take all drugs in the prescribed manner without crushing or mixing them with fruit juice, for example

k. Use such patient education techniques as the following:
(1) Recognizing and addressing language barriers
(2) Using cognitive, psychomotor, and affective learning objectives when teaching
(3) Giving oral and written instructions; e.g., tape pills to a card as a visual aid
(4) Specifying the drug's name and purpose, the method and times of administration, food and activities to avoid or use, information on adverse reactions and procedures to follow if they occur, proper storage method, how long to use medications, and refill procedures
(5) Providing follow-up teaching
(6) Establishing predischarge training programs for managing drug schedules
(7) Teaching individually or in small groups
(8) Designing material that assists with counteracting sensory impairment and memory changes
(9) Using audiovisual aids
(10) Adjusting drug administration instructions to individual life-styles and habits
l. Encourage elderly persons to use assistive devices or special provisions if necessary, including:
(1) Large-print labels on drug containers
(2) Calendars, check-off systems, or commercial devices, such as Mediset, to help remember when to take various medications on schedule
(3) Screw-cap or flip-top containers because childproof containers may be difficult to open
(4) Drugs in liquid form, which may be easier to swallow

G. Exercise
1. General information
    a. The ability to exercise and perform physical work declines with age
    b. Cardiac output declines with age, resulting in decreased maximum work capacity
    c. Vital capacity declines with age, limiting air movement during exercise, which results in an increased respiratory rate
    d. Benefits of an individually prescribed and supervised exercise program include:
    (1) Improved self-esteem
    (2) Increased maximal oxygen uptake, lower heart rate and systolic blood pressure
    (3) Lower serum catecholamine levels
    (4) Reduced adipose tissue and increased percentage of lean body mass
    (5) Increased ratio of high-density lipoproteins
    (6) Improved digestion
    (7) Decreased frequency of constipation
    (8) Strengthening and toning of muscles

(9) Increased cardiovascular function

(10) Increased pulmonary function

(11) Increased interaction and socialization

(12) Increased ability to cope with stress

   e. Lack of physical activity can contribute to poor appetite, constipation, fatigue, insomnia, stress, and depression

2. Contributing factors

   a. Physical activity may be limited from disease processes and pain

   b. Depression and social isolation may contribute to decreased activity level

   c. Elderly persons with temporary or permanent limited mobility from stroke, fractures, arthritis, general weakness, and acute or chronic illness need guidance and encouragement to engage in physical activity

   d. Medications may influence both the elderly person's ability to perform exercise and his physiologic response to it

   e. Other factors that contribute to whether elderly persons exercise include proximity to recreational facilities, income, and their customary recreational activities

3. Possible nursing implications

   a. Keep in mind that the nursing goal is to encourage and assist the person with an exercise program to strengthen muscle tone, improve range of motion and flexibility, relieve boredom, and reduce social isolation

   b. Advise the elderly person to obtain his doctor's approval before beginning an exercise program

   c. Keep in mind any special physical conditions and limitations when designing an exercise program

   d. Monitor the elderly person carefully during any exercise program

   e. Teach the elderly person to watch for such signs and symptoms as shortness of breath, abnormal facial coloring, labored breathing, light-headedness, dizziness, or pain while exercising; instruct him to stop exercising if any of these occur

   f. Caution the elderly person to begin exercise programs slowly

   g. Advise the elderly person to avoid isometric (static) exercises because they stimulate the vagovagal response and raise blood pressure

H. Sleep difficulties

1. General information

   a. Deep sleep (Stages 3 and 4) and rapid eye movement (REM) sleep decrease with aging

   b. Stage 4 sleep has been found to play an essential role in restorative physiologic well-being; REM sleep is necessary for relief of tension and anxiety

   c. The significance of decreased Stage 4 sleep in elderly persons has not been established

   d. Elderly persons normally experience frequent arousals, which may give them a false impression of sleeplessness

     e. Frequent arousals and decreased Stage 3 and 4 sleep cause altered sleep patterns, but the elderly person's need for sleep does not decrease

     f. Napping tends to increase with age and has been shown to provide rest, relaxation, and compensation if less sleep occurs at night

     g. Sleep apnea increases with age and has been associated with cardiac dysrhythmias and sudden death in elderly persons

     h. Hypnotic drugs depress REM sleep

     i. Lack of sleep leads to fatigue, irritability, and increased sensitivity to pain

2. Contributing factors

     a. Minimal environmental stimulation, a change in daily routine, boredom, or extended napping during the day may contribute to insomnia

     b. Persistent physical symptoms, such as leg cramps, pain, coughing, and urinary frequency, may contribute to insomnia

     c. Other factors affecting sleep include nightmares, worry, and bereavement

     d. The most common cause of sleep disturbance in elderly persons is depression

3. Possible nursing implications

     a. Keep in mind that the nursing goal is to promote restful sleep

     b. Begin by assessing and evaluating the person's sleep history, including:

          (1) Current and past sleep patterns

          (2) Changes in sleep patterns

          (3) Napping patterns

          (4) Exercise and activity level

          (5) Diet and use of alcohol, drugs, and caffeine

     c. Educate the elderly person about aging changes and altered sleep patterns

     d. Teach the elderly person to maintain a quiet and restful environment conducive to sleep and to follow usual bedtime rituals

     e. If the elderly person is hospitalized, promote comfort by proper positioning, administering pain medication, and ensuring warmth with enough blankets; maintain the person's bedtime rituals as much as possible

     f. If the elderly person is hospitalized, promote relaxation by giving back rubs or foot rubs and offering warm milk or a glass of wine, if possible

     g. Encourage the elderly person to exercise early in the day to prevent overstimulation at bedtime

I. Leisure-time activities

1. General information

     a. Predictors of retirement satisfaction include general health status and attitudes and feelings about retirement

     b. Preparation for retirement may facilitate adjustment to increased leisure time

     c. Adjustment phases in the retirement process include:

          (1) The retirement event, luncheon, or party usually precipitates exhilaration followed by a letdown

(2) During the "honeymoon" phase the elderly person tries out new activities in order to develop a new life-style

(3) Disenchantment with retirement may follow the honeymoon phase

(4) During the final phase new patterns emerge and develop into a satisfying routine

    d. Leisure activities should be self-determined, pleasurable, and contribute to a sense of self-worth

    e. Choice of leisure activities is influenced by age, health, social network, income, location, work role, and family structure

    f. Changes in health and energy level or impaired sensory function have an impact on the choice of leisure activities

2. Contributing factors

    a. With retirement may come a decrease in income

    b. Retirement may be viewed by some elderly persons as a crisis with the loss of self-esteem they derived from work success

    c. Elderly persons tend to maintain similar patterns of leisure activities throughout life

    d. Elderly persons who have lived a highly structured life-style may experience anxiety with increased unstructured time

3. Possible nursing interventions

    a. Keep in mind that the nursing goal is to assist elderly persons to adjust to increased leisure time

    b. Encourage them to do preretirement planning, including anticipated leisure-time activities

    c. Encourage elderly persons to plan some regular activity outside the home to maintain social interaction and self-esteem

    d. Refer elderly persons to local senior citizen centers and community recreational facilities, if appropriate

    e. Keep in mind that day-care programs may be available for physically or mentally impaired elderly persons

    f. Tell elderly persons about senior citizen groups and organizations that arrange trips and offer discounts; these may particularly interest those who enjoy traveling and socialization

    g. Assist elderly persons who prefer a structured life-style to develop new daily routines

J. Sexual function

1. General information

    a. Sexuality is an important aspect of caring for elderly persons

    b. Sexual interest, activity, and needs are maintained well into old age, provided the individual remains in good health and has an interested and interesting partner

    c. Sexual problems in elderly persons commonly result from emotional or social factors rather than biological or organic conditions

    d. Regular stimulation through intercourse or masturbation helps maintain a person's interest in sex

    e. Arousal may take longer in elderly persons

    f. Sexuality includes such behaviors as touching, kissing, hand-holding, and massages

    g. Intimacy, companionship, and physical nearness are especially important to elderly persons

    h. Sexual function in elderly persons is affected by alterations in erection and ejaculation in men and vaginal lubrication in women

2. Contributing factors

    a. Past sexual activity and enjoyment are the best predictors of sexual behavior in old age

    b. Barriers to sexual expression include poor health, cultural attitudes, opportunity, and the individual's sexual history

    c. Sexual activity may cease because of a partner's illness or death, disinterest, monotony, or substitution of a satisfying nonsexual activity

    d. Fear of failure during sexual intercourse plays an important role in avoiding sexual activity

    e. Illnesses and medications can adversely affect libido and cause erectile problems in older men

    f. A common obstacle to sexual expression among elderly persons is lack of privacy, especially among those living with adult children or in an institution

    g. Common gynecologic problems of older women that interfere with sexual activity include senile vaginitis, vulvitis, perineal pruritus, uterine prolapse, cystocele, and rectocele

    h. Heart disease, especially a history of heart attack, may cause an elderly person to avoid sex from the fear of causing another heart attack

    i. Diabetes may cause impotence in elderly persons

    j. Arthritis may be painful enough to limit sexual activity

    k. Prostatectomy generally does not impair sexual capacity or enjoyment

3. Possible nursing implications

    a. Keep in mind that the nursing goal is to provide information and assist elderly persons in finding their own answers to concerns about sexual function

    b. Help the person become aware of his own beliefs and attitudes about sexuality and aging

    c. Educate elderly persons about the changes in sexual function caused by aging

    d. Assist elderly persons with resolving sexual issues

    e. Incorporate a sexual history in the nursing assessment

    f. Protect and maintain the sexual rights of institutionalized and noninstitutionalized elderly persons

    g. Refer patients with sexual problems for a physical workup and counseling

    h. Advise elderly persons to avoid sexual relations following a large meal, during extremely hot or cold environmental temperatures, in anxiety-provoking situations, or if negative feelings of anger or resentment exist

    i. Recommend position variations for intercourse, such as more passive positions for coronary patients and stroke victims

    j. Offer information about the effect of drugs and alcohol on sexual function

    k. To avoid the negative effects of drugs and alcohol, suggest exercise, rest, and warm baths

    l. Recommend position changes to alleviate joint pain

K. Dental health and oral hygiene

1. General information
   a. Loss of teeth is not a normal part of aging
   b. Tooth loss may result from either tooth decay (dental caries) or impaired supporting structures (periodontal disease)
   c. Periodontal disease, a common problem among elderly persons, causes inflammation that results in degeneration of the tissues supporting the teeth; signs and symptoms include:
      (1) Pain
      (2) Swelling
      (3) Loose teeth
      (4) Fetid breath
      (5) A bad taste
      (6) A fistulous tract
   d. Cumulative factors that contribute to wearing away of teeth over a lifetime include:
      (1) Attrition—grinding from tooth-to-tooth contact, as in chewing
      (2) Abrasion—rubbing away by friction, as from a toothbrush
      (3) Erosion—loss of tooth enamel that results from a chemical process, not from bacteria, as from emesis
   e. It is estimated that one half of adults over age 65 are edentulous
   f. About 90% of oral cancers occur after age 45, usually in men who are heavy smokers or who chew tobacco
   g. Leukoplakia (a precancerous condition) may develop from chronic mouth irritation

2. Contributing factors
   a. Decreased saliva production and drugs that cause dry mouth make elderly persons vulnerable to tooth decay and cause dryness and cracking of oral mucosa
   b. Age-related changes of the oral mucosa (thinning and drying of the epithelium) make older adults more prone to mucosal injury
   c. Some drugs may induce changes in oral mucosa
   d. Decreased sensitivity to the warmth of liquids or foods may cause mouth burns or other oral lesions
   e. Obstacles limiting an elderly person's access to regular dental care include anxiety, unaffordable cost, transportation problems, and lack of a perceived need
   f. Mouth care may not always be part of routine nursing care

    g. Problems associated with dentures include sore mouth, improper fit, difficulty chewing, and inflammatory hyperplasia (tissue flaps around denture edges)

    h. Dehydration contributes to mouth dryness and cracked lips

    i. Breathing through the mouth dries oral mucosa and increases the risk of tissue irritation and damage

  3. Possible nursing implications

    a. Keep in mind that the nursing goal is to prevent tooth loss and periodontal disease by promoting self-care and, if needed, assistance with oral hygiene

    b. Be sure to include oral hygiene as part of routine nursing care

    c. If the patient is unable to perform routine mouth care, clean his mouth with a soft-bristle toothbrush and dental floss to remove plaque

    d. If the patient cannot tolerate brushing or flossing, moisten and cleanse his mouth with normal saline solution; solutions containing alcohol should be avoided

    e. To remove viscous secretions or dried mucus, use sodium bicarbonate (10 cc in 100 ml of normal saline) or hydrogen peroxide solutions ($\frac{1}{4}$ to $\frac{1}{2}$ H_2O_2); be sure to remove these solutions from the mouth with water or saline solution

    f. Teach elderly persons proper brushing and flossing techniques

    g. Educate elderly persons about proper denture care and oral hygiene

    h. Encourage preventive dental care with regular check-ups every 6 to 12 months

    i. Advise elderly patients to remove their dentures at bedtime

L. Nutrition

  1. General information

    a. Many health problems in older adults are the result of poor nutrition

    b. Older persons tend to gain weight more easily because of a decreased basal metabolic rate and reduced physical activity

    c. Although caloric needs are decreased, the recommended amounts of vitamins, minerals, and protein remain essentially the same in old age

    d. Common dietary deficiencies among elderly persons include protein, vitamins C and D, folic acid, calcium, and iron

    e. Nutritional status has an overall effect on health status and energy level

    f. Nutritional deficiencies are usually the result of inappropriate food selections and rarely of inadequate food intake

  2. Contributing factors

    a. Impaired thirst sensation may result in decreased fluid intake

    b. Financial resources may determine the amount of food intake

    c. Ethnic and cultural preferences influence food choices

    d. Immobility may hinder a person's ability to purchase and prepare food

    e. Immobility and lack of exercise contribute to poor appetite

    f. Loneliness and depression can adversely affect eating patterns

    g. Dental problems, such as missing or loose teeth and poorly fitting dentures, affect the person's ability to chew and the types of food that can be eaten

    h. Diminished sense of smell and taste result in decreased stimulation to eat

    i. Impaired digestion from altered stomach or bowel functioning may affect the nutritional status of elderly persons

    j. Institutionalized elderly persons may lose interest in food because of the blandness or monotony of food choices

    k. Complex therapeutic diets may be difficult to understand and prepare, resulting in noncompliance

3. Possible nursing implications

    a. Keep in mind that the nursing goal is to maintain optimal nutritional status through education and diet provisions that incorporate individual preferences

    b. Limit dietary changes to those necessary for health

    c. Educate elderly persons about the use of vitamin and mineral supplements

    d. Teach the principles of good nutrition and explain the rationale for prescribed therapeutic diets

    e. Assist elderly persons with meal planning, keeping in mind cultural and ethnic preferences

    f. Recognize the personal and social aspects of eating meals

    g. Make elderly persons aware of dietary recommendations that may decrease their risk of cancer and heart disease, including:

        (1) Eat more fresh fruits and vegetables and whole grains

        (2) Avoid foods that contain refined and processed sugar

        (3) Decrease consumption of processed foods

        (4) Reduce the amount of fat consumed

        (5) Limit sodium intake

    h. Counsel elderly persons on low incomes to contact their local Department of Social Services to find out if they qualify for food stamps

    i. For elderly persons who live alone, suggest setting an attractive table and preparing an enjoyable meal; the presence of a pet, a good book, or a television or radio program may help them to enjoy their meal more

M. Nursing interventions for common problems among hospitalized elderly persons

1. Poor eating habits

    a. Check whether menu choices have been filled out

    b. If possible, encourage the patient to eat out of bed, or with others

    c. Make sure dentures are in

    d. Have family bring seasonings the patient uses at home; use salt substitutes, if indicated

    e. Provide various of flavorings for dietary supplements and formula feedings

    f. Adjust meals to individual life-styles and daily routines

    g. Be aware that brightly colored foods add interest and variety in meals and smaller portions don't overwhelm the patient

    h. Make sure that trays are served promptly to keep hot food hot and cold food cold

    i. Have snacks, such as toast, custard, hot chocolate, or fruit, available at night

    j. Assist with oral hygiene

    k. Avoid interrupting meals for medications and tests

    l. Offer food substitutions when meals are missed

    m. Make sure the person uses the toilet before eating

    n. Check to see if medications, such as I.V. antibiotics or potassium, are affecting the person's appetite

2. Urinary incontinence

    a. Maintain routines the patient follows at home

    b. Check functional abilities; e.g., whether the patient can get up to go to the bathroom

    c. If the patient uses a bedside commode, make sure he has access to it

    d. After an incontinence episode, ask the patient if he had any forewarning of the need to urinate

    e. Remember that the action of diuretic medications is enhanced when taken by a recumbent patient (because of an increased glomerular filtration rate); plan timing of medication, as appropriate, to promote or prevent this

    f. Consider limiting the amount of coffee, tea, and other stimulants

    g. Limiting fluids after 8:00 p.m. may help

    h. Be aware that the patient will need to void several times a night, more if receiving I.V. therapy

    i. If the patient uses a bedpan, it might be kept in bed for quick access

    j. Keep a bell or call light within reach

    k. Catheterization is used only as last resort

    l. Identify voiding patterns and offer frequent opportunities for using the toilet

    m. Help the patient use the toilet after meals

3. Fecal incontinence

    a. Check for fecal impaction

    b. Check for functional ability; e.g., whether the patient can get up and walk to the bathroom

    c. Check medications; antibiotics may cause diarrhea

    d. Check diagnosis; incontinence may relate to pathophysiology, such as spinal cancer, stroke, or gastrointestinal bleeding

    e. Check for laxative abuse; keep in mind that patients may ask family members to supply laxatives

    f. Check whether the patient is enema-dependent

    g. Institute bowel retraining, if appropriate

    h. Change diet to increase bulk and fiber

4. Constipation
    a. Check for use of narcotics, which can cause constipation
    b. Monitor fluid intake and increase it, if necessary
    c. Suggest drinking hot water with lemon and honey
    d. Incorporate a regular exercise program, if possible
    e. Reestablish previous routines; e.g., bowel movements after meals or first thing in the morning
    f. Make sure water is available and within reach
    g. Give extra fluids with medications
    h. Give juices and other fluids between meals
    i. Check whether the patient's medications can cause constipation
    j. Use a bedside commode instead of a bedpan when possible
    k. Provide uninterrupted privacy when the patient is trying to have a bowel movement
5. Insomnia
    a. Be aware that hospitalization disrupts sleeping patterns
    b. Encourage the use of a night-light, and keep doors to rooms closed
    c. Make sure the patient is warm enough
    d. Decrease noise and other distractions
    e. Make sure the patient uses the toilet before bedtime
    f. Offer a snack
    g. Sit and listen to the patient's concerns
    h. Evaluate whether a roommate change is appropriate
    i. Find out what sleep-inducing measures were used at home; e.g., reading, listening to music, or drinking hot milk
    j. Provide a warm washcloth for the hands and face
    k. Offer a back rub
    l. Assess the patient's need for pain medication
    m. Make sure medications are given before the patient settles down for the night, if possible
    n. Offer the patient more pillows or a more comfortable bed position
    o. Check to see if the patient's medications contain caffeine
    p. Fix sheets and make sure the bottom sheet is smooth
    q. Be aware that the patient may want familiar objects nearby, such as pictures or a clock
    r. Encourage diversionary activity, such as reading or watching television
    s. Help the patient accept the fact that he may have difficulty sleeping
6. Confusion
    a. Use a night-light if confusion seems to happen more at night
    b. Orient the patient to the environment and the equipment in his room
    c. Avoid restraints; instead try using a Geri chair
    d. Ask the family to stay or get someone who can sit with the patient, if necessary
    e. Recognize that the patient may exhibit unusual or inappropriate behavior, such as identifying the nurse as his daughter; accept that what is being said might be meaningful to the patient, but always try to reorient him

    f. Find out whether the patient needs to use the toilet

    g. Place familiar objects where they can be seen

    h. Eliminate or modify pain and sleeping medications

    i. Ask the family how they handle confusion at home and try to adapt these techniques to the hospital environment

    j. Stay calm; staff anxiety makes patients more anxious

    k. Encourage reminiscence, which reduces the patient's confusion as well as his anxiety about being confused

    l. Reduce environmental stimuli

7. Pain

    a. Find out the type of pain; e.g., chest pain, gas, or indigestion

    b. Institute specific interventions when the cause is identified

    c. Keep in mind that multiple causes may exist, but the most frequent cause is musculoskeletal

    d. Get the patient out of bed, and have him perform active and passive range-of-motion exercises

    e. Use warm towels and massage

    f. Use a trapeze to facilitate movement

    g. Have the patient contract and relax each muscle group

    h. Adjust the bed position and pillows

    i. Differentiate pain from discomfort

    j. Look for contributing factors, such as constipation or leg cramps

    k. Try nursing interventions, such as relaxation exercises, before giving sleep medications, if possible

    l. Identify psychological concerns that may make pain or discomfort worse at night; interventions, such as listening, stroking, companionship, or diversionary activities, may help

    m. Get the patient interested in something: television, games, puzzles, reading, or reminiscing

Points to Remember

Falls, burns, hypothermia, fires, and hyperthermia are major safety problems for elderly persons.

Medication misuse is a common problem among elderly patients.

Exercise serves to counteract some problems older adults face, such as immobility.

The aging process alters sleep patterns.

Medications may contribute to sleep disturbances.

Sexual interest and activity normally continue into later life.

Counseling may be necessary to broaden an older adult's opportunities for leisure-time activities.

Nutritional problems may be the direct result of dental problems.

Glossary

Drug absorption—the time required for a medication to enter into general circulation

Drug distribution—the process by which an absorbed drug is transported to organs and peripheral tissues and localized in the tissues

Drug excretion—the process by which a drug is eliminated from the body

Drug metabolism—the sum of all chemical reactions involved in the biotransformation of medications

Leukoplakia—white spots or patches on the mucous membrane of the tongue or cheek that have a tendency to fissure and to become malignant

Pharmacokinetics—the study of drug disposition in the body, including the rate of absorption, distribution, metabolism, and excretion

Sleep apnea—the temporary cessation of breathing during sleep

Resources for Support

Learning Objectives

After studying this section, the reader should be able to:

• State the role that adult children play in caregiving for an elderly parent.

• Describe two community-based services designed to meet the nutrition, housing, or transportation needs of the older adult.

• Describe the major differences between skilled nursing facilities (SNF) and intermediate care facilities (ICF).

• State two reasons why there is a growing interest in home health care.

VIII. Resources for Support

A. Family support
1. General information
   a. The health of the older adult affects relationships, social contacts, care activities, and living arrangements
   b. Illness, hospitalization, and recovery decrease the older person's functional capacity
   c. Loss of functional capacity increases dependence and need for family involvement; role of family members changes as older person ages
   d. Demographic trends show that fewer children are available to share the care of an elderly parent even though the number of four-generation families is increasing
   e. 40% of people in their 50s have a surviving parent and 20% of people in their 60s have a surviving parent
   f. The family unit is the basic social unit and the primary support system for the older adult; besides giving care, families also provide affection and social interaction
   g. Most elderly couples live by themselves, so the spouse is the primary caregiver; children assist with care
   h. If the spouse of the person who needs care dies, children become primary caregivers
   i. Other relatives and friends do not have the duties and responsibilities of the immediate family unit but can act as peripheral, informed caregivers
   j. Although most older adults are independent, one third require help
   k. Older adults prefer to live near, but not with, their children
   l. 84% of older adults live less than 1 hour away from a family member; 18% live with one of their children
   m. Family provides 80% of care of old-old adults
   n. 60% of women ages 45 to 54 and 42% ages 55 to 64 work and are primary caregivers to an elderly person in addition to other roles
   o. Caregiving puts additional physical and mental stress on the family
   p. Physical care puts the greatest demand on a family
   q. Some families cannot and should not be caregivers
   r. Children provide care to prevent institutionalization; many times the functionally impaired older person is maintained at home
   s. In addition to caregiving, adult children have their own health problems, developmental activities, and losses
   t. Caregiver stress results from multiple demands, isolation, loneliness, and low morale; spouse caregiver is vulnerable to health problems from energy drain
   u. Unresolved relationship problems within a family contribute to strain and magnify the crisis
   v. Family members may express guilt and anger; the nature of the older person's health problems may be disturbing

2. Possible nursing implications
   a. Assess the family's ability to act as caregiver
   b. Prepare adult children for shift in dependency as parents age
   c. Recognize interrelationship, independence, and reciprocity of family members' roles
   d. Support elderly person in efforts to maintain autonomy, to participate in care and decision making
   e. Establish a relationship with the family and support all family members
   f. Involve family members in the care of hospitalized or institutionalized older person if they desire
   g. Help family identify and use resources such as respite care and counseling
   h. Teach family members about normal aging process and possible physical and mental problems of elderly parents
   i. Help family members negotiate the sharing of care activities

B. **Community-based resources: nutrition, housing, transportation, and education**
   1. General information
      a. Nutrition
         (1) Federally funded nutrition sites provide one congregate meal per day
         (2) Meals on Wheels delivers meals to homebound
         (3) Church and community groups may provide meals
         (4) Food stamp programs are available to some elderly persons
         (5) Loneliness, rather than lack of money, may create a major nutrition problem for the elderly person because he may not eat properly when alone
         (6) Food programs are designed to improve or maintain nutrition and maintain the elderly person's independence
         (7) Food programs may be based on ability or inability to pay
         (8) Quality of service may determine participation in a food program
         (9) A food program also provides contact with others and an opportunity for relationships
      b. Housing
         (1) 70% of elderly persons live in single homes; 30% live in hotels, rental units, public housing, institutions
         (2) When the elderly person can no longer live in his own home for economic or health reasons, alternative housing choices include age-segregated or age-integrated housing complexes, public housing for elderly persons, shared housing, congregate housing
         (3) Day-care and social programs at community centers that provide care or supervision during the day may prevent a housing crisis by enabling elderly persons to remain at home or with family instead of relocating to an institution
         (4) In rural areas, few alternatives exist and the poorest housing conditions occur

(5) The trend is toward housing alternatives that provide continuity of care, such as life-care facilities

(6) The major factor in housing problems is inadequate income

(7) Many older persons need funds to modify their home so they can remain at home

(8) More support exists for other needs, such as meals, cleaning, transportation, and medication-giving, than for housing

c. Transportation

(1) About 8.3 million people over age 65 drive cars; accidents involving elderly drivers are twice as likely to be fatal as those involving younger drivers

(2) Many older persons depend on friends and relatives for transportation

(3) Transportation problems of elderly persons include lack of a car, inability to drive, economics of keeping a car, distance from such services as health care

(4) Alternatives to driving include reduced-fare taxis, public transportation programs, volunteer drivers, dial-a-ride, and chartered bus excursions

(5) Lack of transportation can lead to social withdrawal, poor nutrition, lack of medical care, and loss of independence

(6) Minority and rural elderly persons are more affected than others

(7) Programs to supplement transportation do not address transportation for pleasure

(8) Volunteers who transport elderly persons may have insurance coverage problems

(9) Public policy considerations include the need for more reduced fares and barrier-free transportation

d. Education

(1) The elderly person can benefit from education because it will build self-esteem, decrease isolation, and maintain intellectual involvement

(2) The elderly person may take or teach classes; relevancy of topic is important

(3) Factors limiting participation include cost, location, transportation, safety

(4) Subjects that often interest the elderly person include health, budget and insurance information, arts, and new skills, such as crafts or home repair

(5) The elderly person may need help with study skills if he decides to pursue a degree

(6) Illiteracy may be a problem

(7) The elderly person usually prefers discovery learning (exploring a topic at one's own pace) because it reduces anxiety and limits evaluation

(8) The elderly person can obtain video and audio cassettes, large-print books from libraries

(9) High schools, colleges, and universities may offer special programs for the older adult that may be for credit or noncredit, short or full-course offerings

(10) The elderly person may qualify for tuition waivers or reduced fees

(11) Elderhostels offer noncredit courses on a live-in basis on residential campus
2. Possible nursing implications for all community-based resources
   a. Assess older person's needs carefully
   b. Know available resources and refer appropriately
   c. Advocate for maintenance and initiation of programs and needs assessment for program development
   d. Assist older person to resolve cost, safety, support issues that may interfere with participation
   e. Keep in mind that community-based programs can meet an older person's needs and prevent institutionalization

C. Acute care resources
1. Hospitals most often provide acute care (the older person can also receive short-term, less intense acute care in the doctor's office)
2. The person must need full-day nursing care to be admitted
3. The focus is on curing and healing
4. The hospital environment results in stress that affects the patient's adaptation
5. Both complex health problems and normal aging changes require adjustments in care
6. The length of stay becomes an economic issue because of the prospective payment system of diagnostic related groups (DRGs)
7. The hospital environment presents cure-versus-care issues for the nurse

D. Long-term care (LTC) resources
1. General information
   a. LTC meets the increasing dependency and support needs of aging persons
   b. No national LTC policy exists
   c. Major problems with LTC include:
      (1) Resource fragmentation and gaps in services
      (2) Multiplicity of funding sources
      (3) Limited number of community-based alternatives to institutional care
      (4) Limited financial reimbursement for care of chronically ill (see Section X)
   d. LTC services provide diagnostic, preventive, therapeutic, rehabilitative, supportive, and maintenance services
   e. LTC services are needed for persons with chronic physical and mental conditions
   f. LTC services are provided in various settings, both institutional and non-institutional
   g. The LTC goal is to promote the person's optimal level of physical, psychological, and social functioning
   h. Use of LTC services is based on medical need, functional status, availability of family and financial support, and the elderly person's living arrangements

    i. The decision about which LTC service to use depends on acceptability, availability, and affordability

    j. Availability of LTC resource is the major determinant of use

    k. LTC reimbursement is a major concern

       (1) LTC insurance is just becoming available

       (2) Medicare and Medicaid reimburse under certain conditions

       (3) Personal financial resources are used to a large extent

    l. Quality of care is a major issue

       (1) Very few registered nurses work in LTC

       (2) Staff receives little education on aging

       (3) Each state sets its own staff requirements

    m. Medicare and Medicaid officials survey facilities

    n. Definitions of the type of facility and programs offered vary from state to state

    o. LTC facilities may be public (government-run), voluntary (non-profit), or proprietary (for profit)

    p. Key differences between LTCs and hospitals include:

       (1) Length of stay

       (2) Type of care

       (3) Perception of quality of care

       (4) Prestige accorded to staff by society

2. Types of institutional LTC

    a. LTC skilled nursing facilities (SNF): nursing homes

       (1) The patient must be chronically ill or disabled and need full-day nursing care

       (2) Physical, occupational, and recreational therapy and social services are available

    b. LTC intermediate care facilities (ICF): nursing homes

       (1) ICFs provide custodial care and personal care services

       (2) The person requires less than 24-hour-a-day nursing care

    c. Home health agencies

       (1) They may be directed by private agencies or hospitals

       (2) Interest in maintaining elderly persons at home is growing for financial and humanitarian reasons

       (3) Fewer home health care agencies and services are available in rural areas

       (4) Many services are limited because of financial reimbursement issues; a national concern

       (5) Medicare and Medicaid strictly limit reimbursable services and do not pay for home services for long-term care; home health care for chronically ill patient is paid for with private resources

       (6) Over 3,000 home health agencies exist

       (7) Home health care provides an alternative to institutional LTC

    d. Other LTC facilities include:

       (1) Rest homes, homes for the aged, convalescent homes

       (2) Range of care from protective environment to personal and some skilled care

    e. Other alternatives to institutional LTC:

        (1) Day care

        (2) Respite care

        (3) Foster care

3. Possible nursing implications

    a. Assist with identifying appropriate level of care

        (1) Assess health and functional status

        (2) Determine range of services needed

        (3) Match resources with need; provide least restrictive environment

    b. Support family decision making

    c. Monitor quality of care using nursing standards and standards of external reviewers, such as Medicare

    d. Advocate for better staff-to-patient ratios in LTC facilities

    e. Plan for transition to LTC facilities

    f. Help family and patient select best LTC facilities, based on the following criteria:

        (1) Amount of privacy available

        (2) Patient and staff relationships

        (3) Types of daily activities

        (4) Patient-to-staff ratios

        (5) Opportunity for family involvement in care plan and activities

        (6) Cost

        (7) Medicare and/or Medicaid certification

        (8) Current licensure

        (9) Medicare and/or Medicaid survey findings on medical, rehabilitative, pharmaceutical, dental, and nutritional services, safety, environment, comfort, and financial status

    g. Use checklist provided by U.S. Department of Health and Human Services for selection criteria; the local health department may assist with referral

    h. Help the elderly person and family explore alternatives for LTC before the need arises

    i. Review statement of residents' rights with elderly person and family, if the facility has such a document

    j. Assist family and elderly person with adjustment to placement

        (1) Family may feel guilty

        (2) Relocation results in stress

        (3) Family and older adult may view placement as the last stage before death

        (4) Placement may represent loss of privacy and control

Points to Remember

Spouses are the primary caregivers for elderly persons.

Families take on additional responsibilities for aged relatives to prevent hospitalization or institutionalization.

The elderly relative's increased dependency on family members creates role reversals.

Community-based programs can provide support to meet needs and postpone institutionalization.

Long-term care provides continuity of care to meet increasing dependency and support needs of aging persons.

Glossary

Congregate meals—group arrangement of meals

Institutionalization—placement of aged person in institutional setting

Protective environment—setting that provides safety and security for elderly person

Respite care—service, offered by some institutions, that provides short-term care of elderly person, thus giving family caregivers a rest

Legal and Ethical Issues

Learning Objectives

After studying this section, the reader should be able to:

• Identify one physical sign, one behavioral sign, and one psychological sign that would cause the nurse to suspect abuse.

• State the four major effects of crime on the elderly person.

• Identify the most restrictive form of protective service.

• State two requirements for a valid informed consent.

IX. Legal and Ethical Issues

A. Abuse or neglect
1. General information
   a. Abuse or neglect is any action or situation that places the elderly person in jeopardy
   b. Abuse or neglect may relate to health status, health care, personhood, right to self-determination, property, or income
   c. Neglect includes failure to maintain safe environment
   d. Types of abuse or neglect include:
      (1) Physical abuse or neglect
      (2) Psychological or verbal abuse
      (3) Violation of rights
      (4) Neglect or omission
      (5) Material or financial abuse
      (6) Sexual abuse or assault
   e. Most likely perpetrators of abuse, in descending order, are:
      (1) Spouse
      (2) Son or daughter, if no spouse exists
      (3) Other caregiver
   f. Abuse or neglect frequently is not reported; elderly person may refuse to file charges; no accurate statistics are available
   g. Abuse may be lifelong pattern or acute response to intolerable situation
2. Characteristics of risk groups
   a. Physical and psychological abuse: white woman, age 66 to 83; not severely ill; income below $7,000
   b. Physical and psychological neglect: white person, age 72 to 89, living with relative; physically dependent; income below $7,000
   c. Financial abuse/neglect: white person age 72 to 89, living with nonrelative; not severely ill; income below $7,000
   d. Person most frequently abused: elderly woman with chronic physical or mental impairment who is perceived as aggressive
3. Signs and symptoms of abused or neglected person
   a. Physical findings
      (1) Unexplained bruises, fractures, or other injuries
      (2) Poor hygiene or grooming
      (3) Malnutrition
      (4) Evidence of inappropriate medication administration
   b. Behavioral findings
      (1) Excessive fear
      (2) Compliant or dependent behavior
      (3) Self-blame
      (4) Avoidance of abuser's touch
      (5) Expressions of concern that abuser is taking person's money or property
      (6) Lack of needed supervision

(7) Lack of money, transportation, or other support to get needed medical care

(8) Inappropriate home maintenance

c. Psychological findings

(1) Evidence of increase in stress and number of crises

(2) Inappropriate coping

(3) Inappropriate expression of anger or guilt in elderly person or abuser

4. Possible nursing implications
   a. Assess typical day's activities
   b. Review history for recent crises and alcohol or drug use
   c. Find out how much outside contact person has
   d. Evaluate person's perceptions of current situation
   e. Assess degree of person's physical, emotional, and financial dependency; also assess availability of shelter from the abuser
   f. Intervene for specific health problems as identified
   g. Make referrals for:
      (1) Community support services such as day care, home health care, and Meals on Wheels, if necessary, to decrease stress on abuser
      (2) Counseling services for all parties
      (3) Social service agencies, such as Adult Protective Services, if available
      (4) Legal services, such as Legal Aid Services and American Civil Liberties Union
   h. Keep in mind that most states require health care personnel to report suspected abuse cases
   i. Contact community emergency services
   j. Participate in prevention activities, such as public education and anticipatory guidance for potential abusers
   k. Support increased resources for support activities and respite care and legislation for mandatory reporting

B. Crime

1. General information
   a. Perception of crime incidence far exceeds actual number of crimes
   b. Elderly persons are more fearful of crime than of illness or inadequate income
   c. Elderly persons suffer no greater physical injury or financial loss from crime than do younger persons; however, crime consequences may be more devastating to elderly persons
   d. Physical, financial, and environmental factors associated with aging increase elderly person's vulnerability to crime
   e. Major effects of crime on the elderly person are fear, isolation, loneliness, and feelings of powerlessness
   f. Crimes against elderly persons include personal and household larceny, household burglary, vehicular theft, assault, robbery, fraudulent schemes, purse snatching, pick-pocketing, and rape

    g. Fraudulent schemes include medical quackery and unreliable or unethical home repair persons, salespersons (including insurance salespersons), and other businesspersons

2. Characteristics of risk group
   a. Personal crime: men age 60 to 70, minorities, unmarried persons, and those with a yearly income below $5,000
   b. Property crime: persons age 65 to 75, minorities, and those living in large communities
   c. Income and location more significant factors than age
   d. Victims age 40 to 65 more likely to be injured during criminal attack
3. Possible nursing implications
   a. Teach the elderly person to know and use available community services, such as escort services, block watch, neighborhood protective networks, and others, to decrease fear and combat isolation
   b. Be aware that Law Enforcement Assistance Administration helps crime victims and that a representative of the Office of Community Victim Assistance Programs can be present at hospital or police station to help victim; this person can also teach elderly persons about crime prevention
   c. Refer elderly person for crime prevention programs and community safety inspections directed at increasing security-conscious behavior, establishing security procedures, and obtaining security devices
   d. Help person identify ways to decrease vulnerability
   e. Encourage person to have Social Security checks mailed directly to bank to decrease risk of mugging
   f. Advocate preventive programs, victim assistance programs, and establishment of community resources

C. Protective services

1. General information
   a. *Adult protective services* is general term for services provided to protect an incompetent person from harm arising from inability to care for self or manage daily affairs
   b. Goal is to provide protection with minimal disruption of life-style and with least restrictive care alternatives; balance freedom with safety
   c. Some communities have an Adult Protective Services agency offering wide range of medical, legal, and social services
   d. Protective services needed by elderly person may include:
      (1) Social support
      (2) Housing assistance
      (3) Support with activities of daily living
      (4) Legal aid
      (5) Financial support
      (6) Medical and personal care
      (7) Emergency services
   e. Types of protective legal arrangements include:
      (1) Power of attorney: legal device whereby older person designates

another to manage affairs; person must be legally competent to initiate this action

(2) Joint tenancy: legal device allowing either elderly person or person having power of attorney to manage the former's affairs

(3) Intervivos trust: trust created by elderly person in which that person serves as first trustee and names successor as second trustee

(4) Conservatorship: designation of a person or institution to take over and protect interests of person judged to be incompetent; court appoints conservator after investigation of person's competence; most restrictive form of protective service; person no longer has right to vote, manage money, determine residence, or make other major decisions; most conservatorships are created for persons over age 75; petition for conservatorship made by family or institutions

(5) Informal guardianship: nonlegal arrangement made with neighbors, nursing homes, private attorneys, banks, trust companies, and nonprofit corporations

  f. Protective rights of elderly persons

(1) Adult has right to make own decisions unless he delegates responsibility voluntarily or court grants responsibility to others

(2) Adult can choose to live in harmful or self-destructive situation provided he is mentally competent, does not harm others, and commits no crime

(3) Rights of long-term-care patient include contract rights; rights of association and communication; rights of autonomy, privacy, and security; rights related to admission, transfer, or discharge; and civil and humanitarian rights

  g. Problems related to protective rights

(1) Competency issue: affluent persons commonly are perceived as eccentric rather than incompetent; poor persons are more likely to be perceived as incompetent

(2) Person may be competent in certain areas but incompetent to make complex decisions; not identifying specific areas of competency leaves aged person at risk of being perceived as incompetent

(3) Informal guardianships have been perceived as having little benefit to elderly person because of purported poor management and abuse

(4) Limits of protective services are determined by degree of protection needed; person who has been judged incompetent to manage own affairs may be seen erroneously as incompetent in all areas

2. Possible nursing implications

  a. Assess and screen areas of competency carefully; assessment has legal, economic, and self-determination consequences

  b. Refer client and family for protective services, when necessary

  c. If informal guardianship has been established, make sure client understands rights and knows which rights have been suspended

  d. Report observations of client's capacity to manage daily affairs

D. Informed consent
   1. General information
      a. Adult must give consent for procedure or treatment unless he has been judged incompetent; guardian must give consent for adult who has been judged incompetent
      b. Institutionalized person has same rights as others but, in some cases, is unjustly denied right to consent
      c. To give valid consent, elderly person must be:
         (1) Fully informed of all risks and benefits of procedure or treatment
         (2) Competent
      d. Federal Department of Health and Human Services also mandates informed consent and human subject review before persons can participate in research
         (1) Guidelines establish informed consent procedures and monitor risk–benefit ratio in studies using human subjects
         (2) In research involving incompetent patient, investigator must obtain permission from appropriate authority; such research is subject to strict review
   2. Possible nursing implications
      a. Assess and screen areas of client competency carefully
      b. Be aware that consent is needed before any treatment, surgical or invasive procedure, and many other procedures and treatments (depending on individual facility) can begin
      c. Follow legal requirements and facility's specific procedures when obtaining client's consent
      d. Follow federal guidelines for consent when client participates in research

E. Quality of life and ethical issues
   1. General information
      a. Quality of life decisions involve weighing risks of diagnostic testing and treatment against chance of benefit and maintenance or enhancement of quality of life
      b. Various factors affect quality of life
         (1) Advances in diagnostic techniques; e.g., echograms, scans, cardiac catheterization
         (2) Advances in treatment; e.g., surgical cures, joint replacement, transplants, cryosurgery, microsurgery, chemotherapy, radiation therapy, life-support techniques
         (3) Increased risk, cost, and, in some cases, questionable benefit associated with these techniques
         (4) Increased data base from which to make decisions because of specialization and development of science and technology; multiple variables must be considered in decision making
      c. Ethical issues occur in care situations in which scientific and medical goals may conflict with ethical/humanistic values; examples include:

(1) Initiation or continuation of treatment of terminally ill patient

(2) Withholding of tube feedings for brain-dead patient; also, issue of who should make this decision

(3) Use of costly medical treatments, such as organ transplantation, for the very old person; also, issue of who should make this decision

2. Contributing factors
   a. Medical science can now prevent and cure many diseases
   b. Death from organ failure can be postponed
   c. Persons age 65 and older have greater incidence of heart attacks, cancer, and stroke than do younger patients; curing one disease may not increase quality of life because other chronic diseases may coexist
   d. Many therapies have unknown risk–benefit ratio for elderly persons

      (1) Clinical treatments and research protocols are usually tested on younger age groups

      (2) Long-term survival rates of some therapies with questionable value or high risk are unknown

      (3) Therapies may carry a risk of poor tolerance, unusual reactions, or questionable value
   e. Depersonalized institutional environments complicate ethical issues
3. Possible nursing implications
   a. American Nurses' Association (ANA) Code of Ethics and Professional Standards provides guidelines for resolving ethical questions
   b. Care goals should be negotiated with patient
   c. Ethical rounds help nurses clarify issues and develop approaches to quality-of-life problems
   d. Concepts and principles should guide ethical decision making

      (1) Autonomy: each individual has responsibility for own decisions and actions and right to information on which to base such decisions and actions

      (2) Nonmaleficence: avoidance of inflicting harm

      (3) Beneficence: taking of actions that contribute to others' health and welfare

      (4) Justice: administration of what is fair, good and deserved; e.g., treatment that reflects human worth and dignity
   e. Goal of ethical decision making is to determine action in patient's best interest

      (1) Based on patient's condition and physical and psychosocial history

      (2) Based on predicted outcome of therapies

      (3) Takes into account multiple variables
   f. Patient's decision about care choices should be supported; support family and others involved in care
   g. Ethical dilemmas necessitate communication with and respect for patient and perspective of all team members

F. Right to die
1. General information
   a. Elderly person has right to decide that he does not want to prolong life by extraordinary means
      (1) Advances in technology allow prolongation of life
      (2) Main issue is quality of life versus length of life
      (3) Anticipatory discussion with patient and family is involved
      (4) Client makes decision after consulting doctor and other health team members
   b. Right to die is an ethical and legal decision; some states have right-to-die laws and legislation, such as living wills (time-limited, patient-initiated, legal method for addressing issue)
   c. Supportive care is continued after decision has been reached
      (1) Such care preserves dignity and comfort, such as skin care, bowel and bladder management, mouth hygiene, and supportive care for patient and family
      (2) Such care limits specific treatment
   d. Factors influencing decision include:
      (1) Patient's suffering
      (2) Patient's cognitive impairment
      (3) Patient's and family's expressed wishes
      (4) Prognosis
      (5) Quality of life
      (6) Current care setting
2. Related issues
   a. Patient's competency to make decision
   b. Family's view of patient's decision
   c. No-code and no-treatment situations
      (1) "Do not resuscitate (DNR)"
      (2) "Do not hospitalize (DNH)"
      (3) "Do not treat (DNT)"
      (4) Doctor's signature required for DNR, DNH, and DNT orders
      (5) Occur more frequently in nursing homes
   d. Euthanasia: painless death that can occur in two ways
      (1) Active: helping someone die
      (2) Passive: permitting death by not actively interfering with natural process
   e. Legal protection provided only when doctors and hospitals follow appropriate policies and procedures
3. Possible nursing implications
   a. Support patient and family in decision making
   b. Support nurses and doctors who implement policies
   c. Ensure that supportive care is maintained

Points to Remember

In most states, abuse is a reportable offense.

The greatest effects of crime on elderly persons are fear, isolation, loneliness, and feeling of powerlessness.

A conservatorship is the most restrictive form of protective service.

The nurse has a major advocacy role in helping clients maintain their right to informed consent.

Determination of a client's competency status and functional abilities has legal, economic, and self-determination consequences.

Glossary

Abuse—misuse or maltreatment that places a person in jeopardy

Competency—ability to perform certain acts and take responsibility for them

Neglect—failure to give proper care or attention

Perpetrator—one who carries out or commits an act

Economics and Health Care

Learning Objectives

After studying this section, the reader should be able to:

● Identify special concerns that elderly persons may have about work and retirement.

● List Social Security Administration programs that provide income and health care for the elderly poor.

● Name major sources of income for the older adult.

● State the difference between Medicare part A and Medicare part B.

X. Economics and Health Care

A. Economy and aging

1. Factors influencing economy
   a. Demographic changes
   b. Social and economic policies affecting elderly person's choices regarding retirement; this, in turn, affects the economy
   c. Changes in retirement patterns, which affect the Social Security Administration's deficit
2. Factors contributing to problems in financing social welfare programs
   a. Changes in economic conditions
   b. Higher unemployment rates
   c. Rapid inflation
   d. Lower productivity
3. Economic resources available for elderly persons
   a. Public financing through taxation
   b. Private income and savings

B. Work and retirement

1. Age of retirement affects work force
2. More people are retiring earlier and living longer
3. Private pension plans may include written provisions that encourage early retirement
4. Decreased income commonly accompanies retirement
5. Inflation makes saving for retirement difficult
6. Factors affecting an elderly person's employment include:
   a. Age discrimination
   b. Potentially reduced competence
   c. Job "burnout"
   d. Physiologic decline
7. Work force is aging
   a. It now includes a higher proportion of older persons
   b. Older workers who stay in the same positions limit others' movement into entry positions and upward mobility
   c. In 1978, Amendment to Age Discrimination in Employment Act raised mandatory retirement age from 65 to 70
   d. In 1985, more than 50% of workers age 65 or older worked part-time
   e. In 1981, 14% of the labor force was age 55 or older
   f. In 1981, less than 3% of the labor force was age 65 or older; three of every five persons in this group were ages 65 to 69; 14% were over age 75

Income and retirement

C. 1. Government income maintenance policies
   a. Policies were developed within current economic framework
   b. Social Security legislation was enacted in 1935

(1) Law provides a continuing income to individuals when their job earnings stop or decrease because of retirement, disability, or a spouse's death

(2) Benefits come from Social Security tax paid by employees, employers, and self-employed workers

(3) Eligibility is based on work credits earned under Social Security

(4) Social Security benefits are based on amount worker paid from earnings over a period of years; government formula determines amount

(5) Social Security benefits include retirement checks (when an individual retires); disability checks (when a worker becomes seriously disabled); survivor's checks (when a worker dies, a survivor's check goes to certain members of his family)

(6) Social Security benefits are also paid to certain dependents of workers who are retired or disabled or who have died

(7) Social Security benefits are intended to provide income protection, not to replace all lost earnings

(8) Retirement income ideally includes a combination of Social Security benefits, pensions, investments, private savings, and other sources

(9) Benefits are periodically adjusted for inflation

c. Welfare programs

(1) Government programs; ensure that individuals can maintain a predetermined standard of living

(2) Eligibility requirements; include income and assets that fall below specified levels

(3) Eligibility based on economic status, not age

(4) Blind, disabled, elderly persons, and mothers with dependent children are usually eligible

(5) Supplemental Security Income (SSI): food stamps, social services, and Medicaid programs included

(6) Supplemental Security Income: a federal program that is state administered; ensures a minimum monthly income to needy people with limited income and resources and who are age 65 or older, blind, or disabled

(7) Food stamps: eligibility varies from state to state

(8) Social services programs: Older Americans Act of 1965; authorized funding for services to elderly persons, with emphasis on maintaining such persons in the community; Administration on Aging channels funds to states, communities, and nonprofit organizations; services channeled through state and area agencies to coordinate delivery of services in community; information about services available at local agencies on aging

(9) Medicaid: Title 19 of the Social Security Act; a joint federal-state program that pays doctor, hospital, nursing home, and other related health costs of eligible poor persons; eligibility requirements vary from state to state

d. Pensions
 (1) Pension regulations have been established by the government
 (2) Preferential tax treatment is given to retirement savings
 (3) Pension fund must be insured by Pension Benefit Guarantee Corporation (U.S. Department of Labor) to protect against bankruptcy of employer and to qualify for tax breaks
 (4) Employee Retirement Income Security Act (ERISA) of 1974 required employers to establish vesting standards
 (5) Federal Civil Service Retirement System includes executive, judicial, and legislative government employees
 (6) Separate retirement pension systems exist for employees of Federal Reserve System, Tennessee Valley Authority, and armed forces
 (7) Separate retirement pension systems exist in most states for state and local government employees
2. Personal income of persons age 65 or older
 a. Purchasing power is affected by personal wealth, continued earnings, government cash, in-kind transfer, and family assistance
 b. Elderly persons have experienced significant improvements in economic status during the last 20 years
 c. Number of individuals age 65 or older with incomes below poverty level fell from 5.5 million in 1959 to 3.9 million in 1980
 d. Gain in earnings has increased savings, thus increasing income available during retirement
 e. Change in median income where female head of household is age 65 or older increased from $3,514 in 1959 to $12,881 in 1980; this represents a real income increase of 40%
 f. Benefits from Medicare, Medicaid, housing assistance, and food stamps programs can increase a single person's income by 32% and a family's income by 14%
 g. In 1985, of those age 65 or older, 21% were at or near the poverty level
 (1) 12.6% of these persons were at the poverty level—11% of them Whites, 32% Blacks, and 24% Hispanics
 (2) 16% of these persons were women; 8% were men
 (3) Single Black women had the highest poverty rate; single white men the lowest
 h. Sources of income include Social Security benefits, asset income, earnings, public and private pensions, and a small amount from other sources
 (1) Social Security benefits are the major source of income
 (2) For approximately 20% of those age 65 or older, Social Security benefits are the sole source of income

D. Health care utilization and health care costs
 1. Health problems of elderly persons are chronic, degenerative, and multiple
 2. Health care system and resources are organized to manage specialty acute care problems, not the chronic, degenerative, multiple health problems of elderly persons

3. Continuity of care between hospitals and community-based primary and rehabilitative care facilities is at best poor; in some cases, nonexistent
4. U.S. health care policy is primarily formulated on assumption that health care is personal responsibility
5. Health promotion and illness prevention may or may not help lower the incidence and onset of chronic disease or reduce degree of disability
6. Government-calculated health care costs do not include cost of assistance from families
7. Elderly persons utilize health care services heavily
   a. In 1984, persons age 65 or older accounted for 31% of total personal health care expenditures
   b. 30% of all hospitalized patients are elderly
   c. Elderly persons accounted for 41% of all hospital days in 1984
   d. Average length of hospital stay of elderly persons is 8 to 9 days
   e. Elderly persons average eight doctor visits per year
   f. In 1984, health care costs for persons over age 65 averaged $4,202
   g. Of elderly persons' health care costs, approximately 45% are hospital expenses; 21% are doctor bills; and 21% are nursing home care
   h. In 1984, 67% of health care costs were covered by government programs

E. Medicare reimbursement
1. Medicare part A
   a. Program was established in 1965 to assist elderly persons with health care costs
   b. Medicare part A covers:
   (1) Inpatient hospital care
   (2) Medically necessary inpatient care in a skilled nursing facility after a hospital stay
   (3) Home health care
   (4) Hospice care
   c. Eligibility is based on individual's Social Security work record or on federal employment
   d. Peer Review Organizations (PROs) consist of group of physicians paid by federal government to review Medicare-related hospital care and investigate patient complaints
   e. Benefits are paid on basis of benefit periods
   (1) Benefit period begins on the first day patient receives Medicare-covered services and ends when patient has remained out of hospital or skilled nursing facility for 60 consecutive days
   (2) Admission to hospital after 60 days begins new benefit period
   (3) Number of benefit periods for hospital or skilled nursing home is unlimited
   (4) Special limited benefit periods apply to hospice care
   f. Medicare part A covers most, but not all, services
   (1) It pays for all covered services for first 60 days of inpatient hospital care in benefit period (except deductible amount—$520 in 1987)

(2) For next 30 days, it pays for all covered services, except $130 per day (in 1987)

(3) If person needs more than 90 days of coverage in given benefit period, 60 reserve days are available; part A covers all but $260 per day (in 1987); reserve days are not renewable

g. Medicare part A covers skilled nursing facility care for skilled nursing and rehabilitation services

(1) Skilled nursing facility must be Medicare-certified

(2) As of 1987, Medicare part A pays for all covered services for first 20 days and pays all costs except $65 per day for next 80 days

h. Medicare part A covers medically necessary home health services

(1) Part-time visiting nurse and physical or speech therapist from Medicare-certified home health agency are covered

(2) Part-time home health aide services, occupational therapy, medical services, and medical supplies may be covered

i. Medicare part A covers hospice care under certain conditions

(1) Maximum of two 90-day benefit periods and one 30-day benefit period

(2) No deductibles or copayments are involved except for outpatient drugs and inpatient respite care

j. Prospective payment system requires hospitals to accept Medicare payments as payments in full and prohibits them from billing patient for anything except applicable deductible and coinsurance amounts plus services and items not covered (such as private television, private duty nurse, or custodial care)

2. Medicare part B

a. Program is a voluntary medical insurance plan; insured party pays a monthly premium

b. Medicare part B covers:

(1) Doctor's services, excluding routine physical examinations

(2) Outpatient hospital care

(3) Home health care, if medically necessary

(4) Physical and speech therapy

(5) Other medical services and supplies that are medically necessary

c. Payments are based on what the law defines as reasonable charges, not by suppliers' current charges

d. As of 1987, patient pays $75 of approved charges; after that, Medicare part B pays 80% of approved charges and patient pays the remaining 20%

e. Doctor, medical supplier, or therapist who accepts assignment of Medicare benefits must accept Medicare's approved amount as full payment and cannot legally bill patient for anything over that amount

f. Doctors and suppliers who agree to accept assignment on all Medicare claims are listed in Medicare Participating Physician/Supplier Directory, available at local Social Security and Railroad Retirement Board offices and at all state and area offices of Administration on Aging

3. Some expenses not covered by Medicare parts A or B
   a. Private duty nursing
   b. Skilled nursing care beyond that covered by Medicare part A
   c. Routine physical examinations
   d. Custodial care
   e. Eye or hearing examinations for prescribing or fitting of eyeglasses or hearing aids
   f. Immunizations, except for pneumococcal vaccinations or other immunizations necessitated by injury or immediate risk of infection
   g. Drugs, other than prescription drugs furnished during hospital or skilled nursing facility stay, or provided by hospice for symptom management
   h. Dental care
   i. Full-time nursing care at home
4. Payments
   a. Medicare benefits change from year to year
   b. Payment system may be confusing to elderly patients, possibly resulting in fear of mishandling bills and checks and difficulty dealing with system
   c. "Patient's Request for Medicare Payment" form (Form 14905) must be submitted to Medicare carrier for payment
   d. Doctor or supplier who uses assignment method of payment or who is Medicare-participating submits claim
   e. Patient submits claim if doctor does not accept Medicare assignment
   f. When submitting claim for rental or purchase of durable medical equipment, patient must include bill from supplier and doctor's prescription indicating type of equipment needed, medical reason, and estimated length of time equipment will be medically necessary
   g. Before payments are made, patient must meet deductible requirement

F. **Private health insurance**
   1. Individual and group health insurance policies vary widely in coverage offered
   2. Types of individual and group health insurance include the following:
      a. Medicare supplement: usually follows Medicare guidelines for services determined to be medically necessary; may pay some or all Medicare deductibles and copayments; some plans are not in best interest of elderly persons, as cost is high and benefits low
      b. Catastrophic or major medical expense: helps cover cost of serious illness or injury, including services not covered by Medicare
      c. Health maintenance organization (HMO): patients pay membership fee or premium and receive services directly from HMO-affiliated doctors and other providers; services are prepaid
      d. Employer group insurance: employer-continued or conversion group insurance
      e. Association group insurance: organizations, other than employers, offering various group health insurance for members over age 65

    3. Medicaid-eligible elderly persons generally do not need additional health insurance

    4. Value and type of additional health insurance should be evaluated on individual basis

G. Possible nursing implications

    1. Recognize cost constraints of elderly person's restricted income

    2. Plan care to contain costs, for example by using:

        a. Generic medications

        b. Community resources

        c. Family resources

    3. Become familiar with current Medicare and Medicaid requirements and limitations of service

    4. Become familiar with community resources

    5. Assist elderly person by providing information and direction in contacting appropriate agencies

    6. Caution elderly person who is considering Medicare supplement (often called Medi-gap) to investigate the program thoroughly; some supplement programs may not be beneficial

Points to Remember

Medicare part A covers hospital expenses.

Medicare part B is a voluntary medical insurance program.

Medicaid is a state-regulated medical assistance program for low-income group.

Billing system for Medicare may be confusing to the elderly person.

An elderly person may need help in dealing with Medicare reimbursement system.

Glossary

Copayment—individual's share of expenses for covered services above deductible amount

Deductible—initial dollar amount not covered by insurance that is paid by individual

Skilled nursing facility—specially qualified facility with staff and equipment needed to provide skilled nursing care or rehabilitative services

Suppliers—persons or organizations, other than doctors or health care facilities, that provide equipment or services covered by medical insurance

The Nurse's Role and Function in Gerontology

Learning Objectives

After studying this section, the reader should be able to:

• Name the American Nurses' Association document that serves as the standard for nursing practice in the care of older adults.

• List the seven ANA standards for gerontologic care.

• Define the nurse's role as advocate for older adults.

• Identify changes in health care delivery that may affect the gerontologic nursing role.

XI. The Nurse's Role and Function in Gerontology

A. Gerontologic nursing roles

1. Practice may be in acute, community, or long-term care environment
2. Practice may focus on elderly patients only or may involve a mixed caseload
3. Growing employment opportunities exist in home health care agencies, wellness clinics, and nursing homes
   a. Persons age 65 or older occupy 60% of all hospital beds
   b. Persons age 65 or older use 60% of all health services
4. Opportunities also exist for specialty practice
   a. Need for specialization, such as in geropsychiatry, long-term care, and education
   b. Need for gerontologic knowledge in other specialties, such as oncology and rheumatology
5. Roles include communicator, planner, case finder, caregiver, comforter, teacher, rehabilitator, and coordinator
6. Multidisciplinary approach is commonly needed in caring for older adult
7. Opportunity exists for challenge and creativity in designing ways to provide quality care
8. Opportunity exists to provide leadership and act as agent for change in altering staff, institutional, and public policy perceptions about aging and health needs of older Americans

B. American Nurses' Association (ANA) Standards of Gerontological Nursing Practice

1. ANA's Division of Geriatric Nursing Practice was ANA's first specialty division to establish standards
2. Standards were issued in 1969; revised in 1976
3. The seven standards address the nursing process and emphasize active involvement of older adult in decision making and goal setting
4. ANA changed term used to describe nursing for older adult from geriatric to gerontological in 1975
   a. Gerontologic nursing represents care and treatment of the elderly person holistically, not just as a diseased or sick person
   b. Geriatric nursing focuses on care of the sick
5. Gerontologic nursing functions include teaching and supervising health maintenance and maximizing individual's biological, psychological, and social resources (See ANA Standards chart)

AMERICAN NURSES' ASSOCIATION STANDARDS OF GERONTOLOGICAL NURSING PRACTICE
Standard I: data are systematically and continuously collected about the health status of the older adult. The data are accessible, communicated, and recorded
Standard II: nursing diagnoses are derived from the identified normal responses of the individual to aging and the data collected about the health status of the older adult

Standard III: a plan of nursing care is developed in conjunction with the older adult and/or significant other(s) that includes goals derived from the nursing diagnosis

Standard IV: the plan of nursing care includes priorities and prescribed nursing approaches and measures to achieve the goals derived from the nursing diagnosis

Standard V: the plan of care is implemented, using appropriate nursing actions

Standard VI: the older adult and/or significant other(s) participate in determining the progress attained in the achievement of established goals

Standard VII: the older adult and/or significant other(s) participate in the ongoing process of assessment, the setting of new goals, the reordering of priorities, the revision of plans for nursing care, and the initiation of new nursing actions

C. Education
1. Undergraduate programs incorporate gerontologic components into basic nursing education
2. Graduate programs prepare nurse to function as gerontologic nurse and gerontologic nurse practitioner

D. Certification
1. ANA certification examination for gerontologic nurse and gerontologic nurse practitioner
   a. Certification is voluntary program
   b. Purpose is to acknowledge professional achievement in nursing
   c. Certification recognizes expertise in applying current knowledge
2. Gerontologic nurse: nurse who is responsible for assessing, planning, and implementing health care for older adult and evaluating effectiveness of care
   a. Baccalaureate degree required
   b. Two years of clinical experience required
3. Gerontologic nurse practitioner: certification examination for nurse prepared in nurse practitioner educational program to deliver primary health services to older adults
   a. 80% to 90% of care problems in nursing homes can be managed by nurse practitioners
   b. To qualify, nurse must have baccalaureate degree and practice experience

E. Gerontologic nursing functions
1. Acute care
   a. Gather medical, family, psychosocial history
   b. Perform patient assessment
   c. Explain diagnosis and treatment to patient and family
   d. Work closely with patient, family, and other professionals to develop nursing care plan

     e. Foster elderly patient's independence
     f. Maintain hydration, nutrition, aeration, comfort
     g. Provide medications and treatment and evaluate response
     h. Inform doctor of change in patient's condition
     i. Administer emergency treatment when necessary
     j. Initiate discharge planning and coordinate referral to community agencies
     k. Serve as patient advocate

2. Long-term care
     a. Gather medical, family, psychosocial history
     b. Perform patient assessment
     c. Involve patient and family in preparation and implementation of nursing plan
     d. Promote an atmosphere that emphasizes living, not disease and dying
     e. Ensure that patient receives medical, dental, podiatric care
     f. Maintain hydration, nutrition, aeration, comfort
     g. Provide medications, treatments, rehabilitative exercises and evaluate response
     h. Teach and advise patient and family
     i. Become knowledgeable about community services for elderly persons and refer patient and family, where appropriate
     j. Inform doctor of change in patient's condition
     k. Perform emergency measures when necessary
     l. Serve as patient advocate

3. Community care
     a. Identify health, social, or economic needs
     b. Refer elderly person to professional or agency best able to meet needs
     c. Explain diagnosis and treatment to patient and family
     d. Evaluate compliance with, and response to, treatment
     e. Use clinic and home visits for health promotion
     f. Teach and advise elderly person and family
     g. Evaluate elderly person's ability to live independently
     h. Become advocate for elderly persons
     i. Encourage elderly person to become advocate on his own behalf

F. Issues affecting gerontologic nursing role
1. Gerontologic nursing research
     a. Nursing studies are needed on clinical problems to improve quality of care
     b. Research areas include cognitive functioning, nutrition, demographic changes, epidemiology, life-style changes, wellness behaviors, sleep patterns, and skin care problems
     c. Studies are also needed on how to adjust or change interventions for older adults
     d. Nursing studies develop gerontologic knowledge by recognizing problems and asking questions; all nurses can participate

2. Advocacy
   a. Definition: representing the interest of another. In part, this can serve to influence institutional, administrative, or legislative policy
      (1) Purpose is to ensure equal opportunity and provide services that a person or certain groups have been unable to obtain
      (2) Nursing definitions include advocacy role
   b. Dynamic process
      (1) Areas appropriate for advocacy may include human rights and responsibilities, ethics, and self-determination
      (2) Advocacy role may include support, information sharing, and working through political channels for benefit of older person
      (3) Nurse assumes active, assertive role as agent for change
      (4) Nurses need to become active in gerontologic nursing organizations, such as ANA's Council on Gerontological Nursing
3. Changes in health care delivery system: prospective payment system
   a. Increasing number of older patients needing services in community results from implementation of diagnostic-related groups (DRGs) and early discharge
   b. More advanced technological services, such as respirators and feeding pumps, can be used at home, enabling patient to leave hospital sooner
   c. Development of prospective payment system for nursing homes may be implemented
4. Development of ANA councils, such as Council on Gerontological Nursing, to set standards
5. Movement of practitioner education into graduate nursing programs
6. Efforts to obtain third-party reimbursement for nurse practitioners
7. Demonstration projects, such as teaching nursing homes

Points to Remember

The gerontologic nurse may practice in acute care, long-term care, or community settings.

The American Nurses' Association has established Standards of Gerontological Nursing Practice.

Gerontologic clinical research is needed to improve quality of care.

Advocacy, a nursing role, involves representing the interests of another.

Glossary

DRG — diagnostic-related group designation, used to set predetermined Medicare reimbursement rates based on classification by patient diagnosis, rather than on charges accumulated during length of stay

Geropsychiatry — psychiatric care of the older patient

Teaching nursing home — nursing home linked with an educational institution for instruction of students and training of doctors and nurses in gerontologic care at the nursing home

Wellness clinics — clinics that specialize in health promotion and maintenance

Appendix

Resources

Government agencies on aging

Administration on Aging
Department of Health and Human Services
330 Independence Ave., S.W.
Washington, D.C. 20201

Architectural and Transportation Barriers
Compliance
  Board
330 C St., S.W., Room 1010
Washington, D.C. 20202

National Institute on Aging
Building 31C
9000 Rockville Pike
Bethesda, Md. 20205

State and local agencies: check your local directory

Health organizations on aging

American Association for Geriatric Psychiatry
P.O. Box 376-A
Greenbelt, Md. 20770

American Geriatrics Society
770 Lexington Ave., Suite 400
New York, N.Y. 10021

American Health Care Association (nursing homes)
1200 15th St., N.W.
Washington, D.C. 20005

American Nurses' Association
Council on Gerontological Nursing
2420 Pershing Rd.
Kansas City, Mo. 64108

American Society for Geriatric Dentistry
211 E. Chicago Ave.
Chicago, Ill. 60611

Gerontological Society of America
1411 K St., N.W., Suite 300
Washington, D.C. 20005

National Association for Home Care
519 C St., N.E.
Washington, D.C. 20002

National Hospice Organization
1901 N. Ft. Myer Dr., Suite 307
Arlington, Va. 22209

Social welfare organizations on aging

American Association of Retired Persons
1909 K St., N.W.
Washington, D.C. 20049

Gray Panthers
311 S. Juniper St., Suite 601
Philadelphia, Pa. 19107

Institute for Retired Professionals
New School for Social Research
66 W. 12th St.
New York, N.Y. 10011

National Center on Black Aged
1424 K St., N.W., Suite 500
Washington, D.C. 20005

National Council on the Aging
600 Maryland Ave., S.W., West Wing 100
Washington, D.C. 20024

National Institute on Adult Daycare
c/o National Council on the Aging
600 Maryland Ave., S.W., West Wing 100
Washington, D.C. 20024

National Senior Citizens Law Center
2025 M St., N.W., Suite 400
Washington, D.C. 20036

Other health and social welfare organizations for the older adult

Alcoholism (check your local telephone directory for local chapters)

Alcoholics Anonymous World Services
P.O. Box 459, Grand Central Station
New York, N.Y. 10163

Al-Anon Family Group Headquarters
1372 Broadway
New York, N.Y. 10018

Arthritis
Arthritis Foundation
1314 Spring St., N.W.
Atlanta, Ga. 30309

Cancer
American Cancer Society
90 Park Ave.
New York, N.Y. 10016

Heart disease
American Heart Association
7320 Greenville Ave.
Dallas, Tex. 75231

Hearing impairment
Alexander Graham Bell Association
for the Deaf
3417 Volta Pl., N.W.
Washington, D.C. 20007

National Association of the Deaf
814 Thayer Ave.
Silver Spring, Md. 20910

National Hearing Aid Society
20361 Middlebelt Rd.
Livonia, Mich. 48152

Kidney disorders
National Kidney Foundation
Two Park Ave.
New York, N.Y. 10016

Mental health
National Mental Health Association
1021 Prince St.
Alexandria, Va. 22314

Respiratory disorders
American Lung Association
1740 Broadway
New York, N.Y. 10019

Speech problems
American Speech-Language-Hearing
Association
10801 Rockville Pike
Rockville, Md. 20852

Stroke
Stroke Club International
805 12th St.
Galveston, Tex. 77550

Vision impairments
American Council of the Blind
1010 Vermont Ave., N.W., Suite 1100
Washington, D.C. 20005

American Foundation for the Blind
15 W. 16th St.
New York, N.Y. 10011

American Printing House for the Blind
P.O. Box 6085
1839 Frankfort Ave.
Louisville, Ky. 40206

Blinded Veterans Association
1726 M St., N.W., Suite 800
Washington, D.C. 20036

Library of Congress
Division for the Blind and Physically
Handicapped
1291 Taylor St., N.W.
Washington, D.C. 20542

National Society to Prevent Blindness
500 E. Remington Rd.
Schaumberg, Ill. 60173

Index

Notes

Notes

Notes

Notes

Notes

Notes

Notes

Notes

Notes